Praise for
Helen Yoest **and** *Plants with Benefits*

🌱

"Filled with little-known secrets, growing tips and titillating tidbits, Plants with Benefits is a must-have catalog of plants that will satisfy all your libidinous botanical curiosities. Good luck not getting emotionally invested."

– James A. Baggett, Editor, Country Gardens

"Plants with Benefits will surely give you a whole new way to look at gardening – for a purpose that everyone can relate to with enthusiasm!"

– Christina Salwitz, The Personal Garden Coach, co-author of Fine Foliage

"Peel back the covers of Plants with Benefits and treat yourself to beguiling photos and tales of flirtatious produce, hot herbs and saucy spices that will tickle your senses and delight your eye. Helen's playful look at the secret lives of her subjects makes for a book that will leave you wanting more! Oh la la!"

– David Spain, Moss and Stone Gardens

"When I heard that Helen was writing a book about aphrodisiac plants, I was delighted! Who better to dig into the secret life stories of the plants in our gardens?"

– Laura Mumaw Palmer, Director, Open Days Program, The Garden Conservancy

"Leave it to Helen Yoest to come up with an intoxicating way to introduce us to a bit of historical (and hysterical) plant folklore. Helen's uniquely euphoric approach will make your day!"

– Nancy Heckler, General Manager, Heronswood

"Helen's passion for horticulture is a feast for the senses. She's a consummate gardener with an uninhibited approach that inspires gardeners to believe the only limits in their garden are their imaginations."

– Chris Sabbarese, Digital Marketing & Communications Manager
Corona Tools

"Helen Yoest's garden writing is nurtured from her lifelong love affair with plants and infused with her down-to-earth humor. Plants with Benefits will introduce you to new ways to use the plants you already have and love. "

– Janet Endsley, Seminar Manager
Northwest Flower & Garden Show

"Helen is one of the rare individuals who combines the eye of an artist with the dirty knees and fingernails of a hands-on gardener. The enthusiasm she has for plants and gardens shows clearly in her writing and speaking, where she distills her personal experience into truly usable advice."

– Mark Weathington, Assistant Director and Curator of Collections
JC Raulston Arboretum at North Carolina State University

Plants
with *Benefits*

Plants
with *Benefits*

An Uninhibited Guide to the Aphrodisiac Herbs, Fruits,
Flowers & Veggies in Your Garden

HELEN YOEST

st. lynn's
press
PITTSBURGH

Plants With Benefits
An Uninhibited Guide to the Aphrodisiac Herbs, Fruits, Flowers & Veggies in Your Garden

ISBN-13: 978-0-9892688-0-6

Library of Congress Control Number: 2013941490
CIP information available upon request

First Edition, 2014

St. Lynn's Press . POB 18680 . Pittsburgh, PA 15236
412.466.0790 . www.stlynnspress.com

Book design – Holly Rosborough
Editor – Catherine Dees
Editorial interns – Allison Keene, Annamarie Mickey, Claire Stetzer and Chloe Wertz

Photo credits:
Ken Gergle – Front & Back Covers, 2, 4, 14, 18, 24, 36, 38, 40, 44, 72, 74, 86, 88, 98, 101, 108, 116, 118, 120, 124, 128, 130, 133
David Spain – 7, 12, 26, 50, 56,
Carolyn Binder – 8, 11, 22, 31, 32, 35, 46, 59, 64, 67, 77, 111
Steve Asbell – 68, 71
iStock Photos – 43, 79, 96, 97, 102
Meredith Corporation – "Photography by Marty Baldwin. Reprinted with permission
from *Country Gardens*® magazine. ©2011 Meredith Corporation. All rights reserved." : 90, 93
JC Raulston Arboretum at North Carolina State University – 106
Holly Rosborough – 112, 126
Helen Yoest – All other photos

Printed in Canada
on certified FSC recycled paper using soy-based inks

This title and all St. Lynn's Press books may be purchased for educational,
business or sales promotional use. For information please write:
Special Markets Department . St. Lynn's Press . POB 18680 . Pittsburgh, PA 15236

10 9 8 7 6 5 4 3 2

To the JC Raulston Arboretum
at North Carolina State University
where I deepened my love of gardening and
plants and learned about right plant, right place.

I've gardened all my life, but I didn't really begin to
learn about plants until I first visited
the JC Raulston Arboretum in 1988.

❦

Plan – and plant for a better world.

~ Dr. J.C. Raulston (1940-1996)

Table of Contents

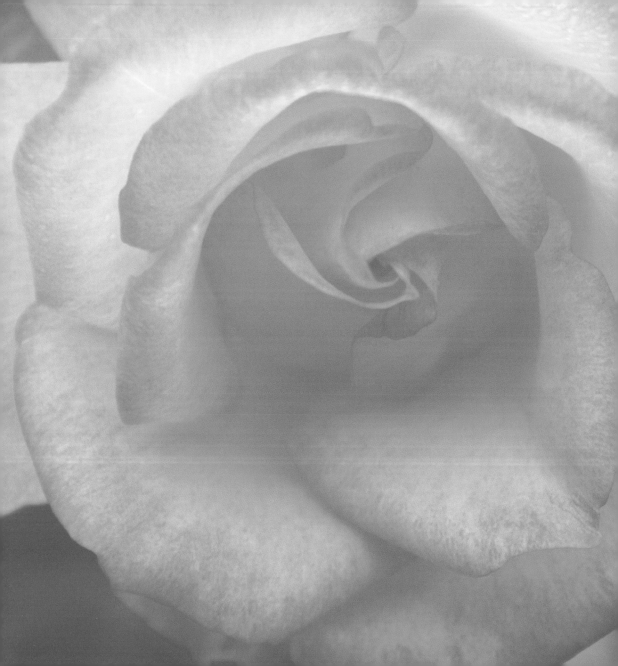

Introduction

I didn't set out to write a botanical *Kama Sutra*. I am a gardener. I write about designing gardens that are in harmony with nature. When I see a plant, I want to know what it does, which of my senses it will satisfy. I'm intrigued by the idea that many plants have a special appeal to one or more of our senses, communicating with us through sight, smell, touch and taste. I think that's one reason some gardens give us such a deep feeling of contentment. So I stay on the lookout for new "sensual" plants to add to my clients' gardens.

That was the book idea I pitched to my publisher, Paul Kelly: creating gardens for the five senses – something I knew quite a lot about. His response was, "Sounds lovely, but with a title like *Plants with Benefits*, aren't you promising a lot more than that?" Well, yes, I suppose I was. And then he said, "Why not go all-out and write a book about aphrodisiac plants?" As he tells it, I paused for a long beat of time before I replied: "Sure...I'd love to!"

So began my quest to understand how plants can play with our erotic feelings, as well as stimulate our sense of wellbeing and receptivity to intimacy. Very soon, it became clear that Mother Nature, in collusion with that sly fellow, Pan, had not only provided us humans with a cornucopia of plants that feed and heal us, but that assure our continual interest in procreation. How did they manage it? As I was to learn, the aphrodisiac effects of certain plants could be subtle – almost subliminal – and they could be blatant; they could arouse a sleeping libido in oh-so-many ways.

Take the banana, for instance: the mere sight of a single banana has arousal tendencies for some of us. (More on that later.) There is no shame in buying a bunch of bananas. On the shelves at the grocery store, clusters of bananas, called hands, are lined up on choir risers for easy inspection and access, singing their own praises – still green, fading verde, solid yellow, or beginning to spot – each humming buy me in a different tune. We choose the hand that will best meet our needs.

Individually, a single banana is called a finger. Once it has been separated from the hand, snapped from the pack and placed into the hand of man, its value can go way beyond its known nutritional benefits and lure us into sophomoric humor, sensual thoughts and even lust. I wondered, was that merely a trick of the highly suggestible human mind? And what about all those other plants that had erotic reputations? You probably know several without my telling.

But I needed to know if there was more to back up these plants' aphrodisiac claims to fame – other than suggestion alone. Was it fable or fact? But then, if it works, does it matter what science says?

In the beginning

Since the deep past of history, aphrodisiacs have been identified and sought out as a remedy for various sexual anxieties and to increase fertility. Procreation being rather important to the continuation of the race, fertility has long been an important moral, religious and societal issue.

Enter the aphrodisiac plants – nature's little helpers.

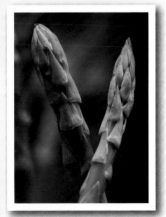

The aphrodisiacs featured in this book have been known to act as catalysts for fertility and, yes, sexual performance due to their physiological and psychological effects. Aphrodisiacs are based on the principle that what a person eats, drinks, rubs on the skin, inhales – or simply views – can have an impact on his or her sex life, whether direct or indirect.

How a plant made the list

As I got seriously into my research, looking for possible explanations for various plants' aphrodisiacal reputations, a pattern presented itself. To make my list, a plant had to have one or more of three qualities that could affect our pleasure centers. But I couldn't ignore the importance of a fourth quality: a plant's ability to increase a person's overall health and vigor.

Quality #1: A plant is psychologically suggestive because of aroma or shape. Sometimes, just thinking that something is an aphrodisiac is enough to make it work as one. If it looks like a duck and walks like a duck...

Quality #2: A plant affects brain chemistry by directly increasing blood flow to sex organs or contributing to other pleasurable sensations.

Quality #3: A plant's hormones mimic human hormones – like a tonic to ignite your own hormones. Researchers are finding that some foods do stimulate the production of hormones that affect our libidos. What they don't yet know is whether those hormones are present in a high enough quantity for us to really notice the difference. Coriander is a case in point.

Quality #4: A plant promotes health and vigor. We know that good nutrition is linked to good health and high energy levels – which admittedly can help set the stage for an active sex life. On that basis alone, hundreds of healthy foods would have made the list for this book; however, I limited my plant list to ones that had an aphrodisiac history.

The Food and Drug Administration is leery of endorsing aphrodisiac claims for plants. But, as we will see, the sheer weight of tradition and anecdotal evidence – aided by some intriguing confirmations from science – tells a different story.

On the non-governmental side of science, psychiatrist Alan R. Hirsch, M.D., F.A.C.P., has conducted and published more than 200 research studies on the effects of smell and taste on human emotions and behavior. As Neurological Director of The Smell & Taste Treatment and Research Foundation, he has found that certain plant-based foods do indeed increase sexual arousal. We'll encounter Dr. Hirsch's research here and there on these pages.

Can a plant's purpose be read, like a book?

In ancient times, there was the Doctrine of Signatures, a philosophy shared by many modern herbalists. The Doctrine was based on the idea that plants that in some way resemble various parts of the body can be used to treat ailments of that body part. These ailments included issues with male and female reproductive organs and libido. In its purest application this was no shallow "magical thinking," but was grounded in great subtleties of observation. The 1st century Greek physician and botanist Dioscorides taught the Doctrine, as did Galen, the greatest physician of ancient Rome; and Paracelsus, the storied Renaissance physician. Not to mention the shamans of the world's indigenous cultures, many of whom are today teaching visiting botanists how to "read" the healing signatures of plants. Some in modern science agree that signatures can provide accurate information, while others find the signatures famously flawed, simplistic and naive.

With all of this in mind, I returned to my consideration of bananas. Why, in some quarters, were they the poster child for desire? Rich in potassium, bananas are certainly good for you, and we know that low potassium can negatively affect sex drive. However, if you were looking for more potassium to increase your performance, you should reach for a sweet potato, an orange, beet greens, or white beans first. Each of these has significantly more potassium than the banana.

Could it be the vitamin B in a banana, then? Vitamins B3, B6, and B12 all work in ways to increase your libido – though, if you need to increase these vitamins, you could instead eat more liver, halibut, and pork chops; or you could take a pill from the health food aisle. Yet, we reach for a single banana instead, for it also puts a grin on our face.

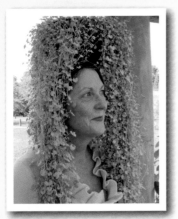

Maybe the good doctors and philosophers of our forefathers should have called these botanical mysteries Signatures of Desire. A plant that helps us to love is a plant worth having. Whether grown in our gardens or purchased at the market, there are indeed plants with benefits – ones that encourage our feelings of intimacy and help us fulfill desire.

Plants with Benefits explores these wonders in nature, plants that can set a romantic stage, be it lore or illusion, fact or fiction. Come, let's discover what others have known for centuries.

Helen

The Plants

Almonds ❧ *Prunus dulcis*

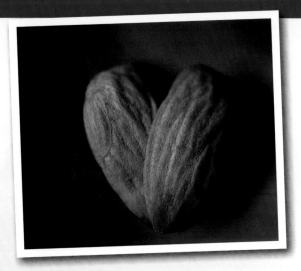

What's all the **female arousal** talk about?

*A*LMOND'S ALLURING SCENT WAS PROBABLY THE GATEWAY BENEFIT FOR THIS reported aphrodisiac. The story since ancient times is that the aroma arouses passion in females. Ladies, if you aren't getting the feeling by smelling the nut (actually a drupe), try taking a whiff of almond in a paste or marzipan form, or even a cookie; it can drive you, well, nuts!

Almonds were domesticated by at least 3,000 B.C., and perhaps earlier. Wild almonds have been found in Greek archeological sites dating back to 8,000 B.C. One of the oldest known aphrodisiacs, almonds symbolize fertility. In the Bible, we read of Sampson wooing Delilah with almond branches, poor fellow. And later, we find the Romans showering newlyweds with almonds, hoping to get the young couple off to a good start.

It's also been said that the French writer Alexandre Dumas, author of *The Count of Monte Cristo*, dined on almond soup each night before hooking up with his mistress. I suppose he

ALMONDS

Family: Rosaceae

Type: Deciduous tree; showy, edible fruit

Color: Rich brown

Harvest Period: Fall

Size: 10 to 15 feet high and wide

Soil: Not picky, as long as alkaline pH is met.

Exposure: Full sun

Watering: Medium

pH: 7 to 8.5

Cold Hardiness Zone: 7 to 9

Origin: Western Asia, Pakistan to the Mediterranean

Why It Works: A Closer Look

While many women love the scent, and probably wondered what was going on whenever they got near marzipan, almonds do provide a high dose of B vitamins, vitamin E, magnesium, and zinc as well as essential fatty acids, which are needed for the production of hormones, reproductive function, fertility, and a healthy libido. Almonds also contain amino acids such as L-arginine which is known to increase arousal. How many almonds would you need to eat to put this amino acid in action? My exhaustive research hasn't given me a number, but no matter – almonds are a good healthy snack, leading you in the right direction. ✄

thought the scent would carry him through the evening. In my hopeless romantic heart, it did.

Cashing in on the scent. Almonds and almond flowers are what all the female-arousal talk is about. Marketing got the memo too, since there is an abundance of almond-flavored oils, soaps, lotions, and potions targeted at us women. I take no offense to that because, um, I really do like the smell.

GROWING TIPS

While an almond tree will grow in mild climates, there can be problems getting it to fruit if there are late freezes. Almonds do better in moderate to warm climates. Even so, almonds are susceptible to a large number of insect and disease problems. It might be in your best interest to purchase your almonds instead of trying to grow a tree yourself. Unless of course you live in California, which is a veritable horn of plenty when it comes to fruits and nuts.

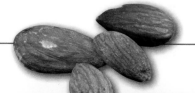

Anise, Aniseed ⚘ *Pimpinella anisum*

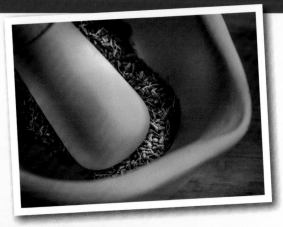

Seeds of desire

*𝒪*F YOU CAN BELIEVE SOME HISTORIANS (AND THE MOVIES, AND A CERTAIN VILLA at Pompeii), Greek and Roman cultures were hotbeds of sexuality. While these sexual practices are likely exaggerated, they nonetheless have a "scandalous" reputation. It's possible, though, that our ancient Mediterranean friends just had a healthy libido, made even healthier by some of the foods they consumed.

Case in point. Anise (or aniseed), *Pimpinella anisum*, was used as both food and aphrodisiac during Classical times. Pliny the Elder and the physician and botanist Dioscorides recorded its use in flavoring foods and wine. Popular lore had it that you could increase desire by sucking on the seeds of this annual herb.

Why It Works: A Closer Look

There is some science behind the lore. Aniseed contains anethole, a phenylpropene that imparts anise's distinctive flavor. For many of us, its aroma and taste alone are enough to increase arousal. But there's more. On the aphrodisiac side, anethole has estrogenic properties

4

ANISE, ANISEED

Family: Apiaceae

Type: Annual herb

Color: Dried seeds are a brown color

Harvest Period: Gather seeds in the fall when they start to turn brown. Cut the umbel flower stalk and hang upside down in a dry location for about a week.

Size: 18 inches to 2 feet tall

Soil: Sandy soil to fairly rich soil

Exposure: Full sun

Watering: Dry to moist

pH: 6 to 7.5

Cold Hardiness Zone: Zone 8, frost tender, annual

Origin: Anise is native to the Mediterranean region, particularly Egypt, Greece and Asia Minor, but it is cultivated widely throughout the world, notably India and South America. *Note:* not be confused with a more familiar-looking seed known as Star Anise *(Illicium verum),* which is actually a member of the magnolia family and not a true anise.

known to stimulate sexual drive by inducing effects similar to testosterone. A 2008 study of anise showed that the essential oils in its seeds and leaves are 90% anethole.

Anise leaves can be eaten raw for a refreshing chew or used to perk up salads, soups and stews. If you're using anise to season your dishes, though, make sure you add it in the last few minutes of cooking, or you'll lose much of its flavor. As for the seeds, you'll find their anethole-rich oil extract used in various sweets, pickles, and teas – in Indian and European cuisines, and in drinks like anisette, pastis, Pernod and ouzo. The notorious spirit absinthe is also flavored with anise (see next page). ✄

GROWING TIPS

Propagate anise seed through direct sowing as early in the growing season as possible. You'll need a long, hot summer to get a decent seed harvest. But here's some good news – if your summers aren't hot enough (or long enough), the seeds are readily available for purchase.

Harvest the ripe seeds by cutting the whole plant and drying it upside-down in a hot, dry location for about a week. Then store the seeds in an air-tight container, ready for use!

Absinthe

an anise-flavored spirit

Once the cocktail of choice in Paris' wealthy nightclub scene – and even outlawed in the early 1900s as a notorious elixir that made men go mad – absinthe is now enjoying a comeback. The classic ritual that goes with this cocktail is part of the fun – and the mystique (instead of a shot, you pour a dose, to give it a dangerous allure).

INGREDIENTS

Absinthe

Absinthe spoon (flat and perforated, preferably silver and ornate)

Sugar cube

Ice water

(The absinthe to water ratio should be from 1:3 to 1:5)

THE RITUAL

Pour a dose into a glass.

Place the sugar cube onto the spoon and rest the spoon on the rim of the glass.

Very slowly, drip ice water onto the sugar cube, drop by drop, until the sugar cube dissolves into the glass. Follow with a thin stream of the remaining water.

Watch intently as the absinthe gradually begins to turn from green to an opalescent white.

Drink slowly, with smoldering eyes.

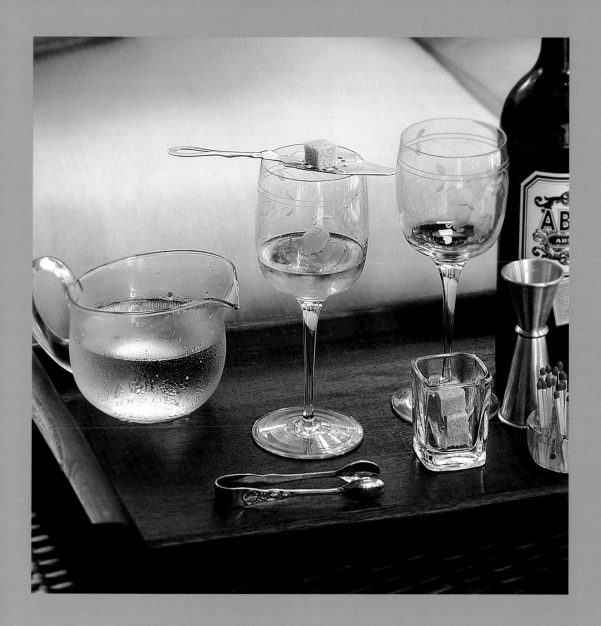

Arugula ✌ *Eruca vesicaria sativa*

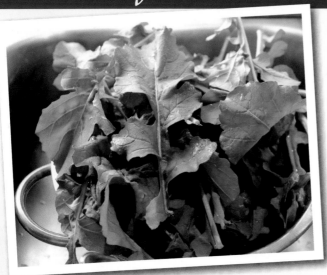

aka:
The Rocket...
enough
said

𝒯HOUGH THE BITTER TANG OF ARUGULA'S OAK-SHAPED LEAVES MIGHT BE TOO spicy for your palate, its aphrodisiac effects might just have you reaching for that second bite anyway.

Ancient appetites. Native to the Mediterranean region, arugula (also called rocket) was historically eaten during meals for its natural aphrodisiac benefits. It was documented as early as the 1st century A.D. by Pliny the Elder and Dioscorides, who cited its ability to increase libido, along with its other health benefits. Arugula was thought to clear the mind while increasing power and energy. Virgil wrote of it: "The rocket excites the sexual desire of drowsy people." This may have led the Romans to consecrate arugula to Priapus, that extraordinarily well-endowed god of fertility and protector of gardens and domestic animals.

ARUGULA

Family: Brassicaceae

Harvest Period: Cool season crop; harvest leafy greens in spring before it bolts, or flowers and seed after bolting.

Color: Dark leafy green

Type: Annual cool-season vegetable, will naturalize

Size: 2 to 3 feet high; 12 to 18 inches wide

Soil: Average, well-drained soil

Exposure: Full sun to partial shade

Watering: Moist

pH: 6.5

Cold Hardiness Zone: Annual. Will take a light freeze.

Origin: Arugula is native to the Mediterranean region, from Morocco to Lebanon.

Why It Works: A Closer Look

As an excellent source of chlorophyll, it can cleanse and energize the blood by providing oxygen to all parts of the body, including your genitals. Today, it's believed that the most important benefit of arugula is improving the quality of blood. It contains high amounts of vitamins K and P, which enhance the function of the liver and absorb calcium. Although arugula is not a direct libido enhancer as the Greeks and Romans supposed, it is rich in A, C, and iron, plus trace minerals and other antioxidants that not only protect against cancer, but also block libido-reducing environmental contaminants from your body.

Despite the lack of modern evidence for arugula's aphrodisiac affects, adding this spicy plant to your diet may make you feel better overall, and that alone is a lure to a questing libido. ✄

GROWING TIPS

Arugula is a cool-season annual in the Brassicaceae family. In the fall or early spring (depending on your location), directly sow arugula seed in a prepared bed. Arugula likes cool weather and can even withstand a light freeze, but will bolt (sending up a flowers stalk and going to seed) when the weather warms. Once this happens, the leaves aren't as tender or flavorful, so harvest the leaves when they are young and small.

Generally speaking, the larger the leaf, the more bitter-tasting the herb, so if you do let arugula bolt, the bitter flowers will make a nice garnish to salads. If left to seed, arugula will self-sow for a continual harvest, at least until conditions become too hot.

Arugula Salad with Honey Pecan Vinaigrette

From the kitchen of
Carolyn Binder,
Cowlick Cottage Farm

This sultry salad has several aphrodisiac ingredients, with arugula topping the list. The bitter taste of arugula is softened with the sweet taste of the honey pecan vinaigrette.

INGREDIENTS

A package or bunch of washed arugula
Crumbled Feta cheese, for garnish
Candied cranberries, for garnish
Chopped shallot or red onion,
for garnish

The vinaigrette:

¼ cup minced shallot or red onion
2 cloves garlic, minced
¼ cup balsamic vinegar
1 tablespoon Dijon mustard
⅓ cup honey (preferably local)
½ teaspoon salt
½ teaspoon black pepper
1 cup extra virgin olive oil
½ cup roasted pecans, chopped

PREPARATION

Combine all the dressing ingredients in a jam jar. Shake well to blend and emulsify. Place arugula in a serving bowl, add Feta, cranberries and shallot or onion. Drizzle with desired quantity of vinaigrette, toss and serve.

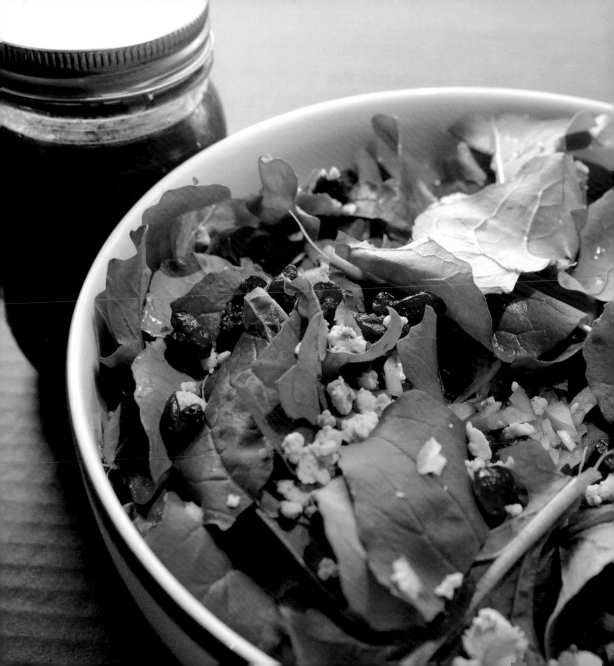

Asparagus ❧ *Asparagus officinalis*

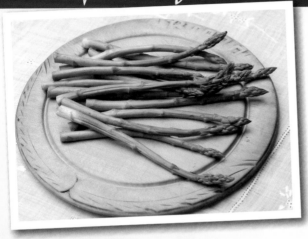

A shape that speaks for itself

THE 17TH CENTURY ENGLISH HERBALIST, NICHOLAS CULPEPPER, WROTE THAT asparagus "stirs up lust in man and woman." And if you were a male in the 19th century France, your prenuptial dinner included three courses of this sexy spear. They couldn't have known it at the time, but asparagus is rich in folic acid, which is said to boost histamine production necessary for the ability of both men and women to reach the big O.

As early as 200 B.C., Cato educated others on growing asparagus. Later Romans, including Pliny, Julius Caesar and Augustus, held the wild variety in high esteem. In the meantime, the ancient Egyptians were cultivating it, selecting out ever-bigger and better varieties.

In Ayurvedic medicine (a system of traditional and alternative medicine found in ancient Indian culture and widely practiced today), *Asparagus racemosus* was recommend for the treatment of gastric ulcers, dyspepsia (indigestion), and as a galactagogue (promoting breast milk production) enhancer. And it was reported to also help with nervous disorders; perhaps the sexual overtones of this phallic-shaped vegetable lightened the mood.

ASPARAGUS

Family: Asparagaceae, formally with Liliaceae

Type: Perennial vegetable

Color: Mostly dark green, but some other colors

Harvest Period: April – May. Roots take 2 to 3 years to produce a crop.

Size: 1 to 3 feet high, 3 to 6 feet wide

Soil: Organically rich

Exposure: Full sun to part shade

Watering: Medium moisture

pH: 6.5 or higher

Cold Hardiness Zone: 4 to 8

Origin: Eastern Mediteranean and Asia Minor areas.

Might I suggest? Foods we consume can have a direct impact on our sex life, whether it's from affecting our hormones, altering brain chemistry, increasing energy or reducing stress levels. Then there are foods that simply suggest sex, and these cannot be ignored.

The asparagus that first became the suggestive aphrodisiac was the wild asparagus, *Asparagus racemosus*, and not the cultivated form we eat and grow today, *Asparagus officinalis*. Both, however, look like little, earthy erections. Imagine one's reaction when first coming upon a field of wild asparagus during early spring growth. Words fail me.

Why It Works: A Closer Look

No doubt, the asparagus is a psychologically suggestive food. But on the biological side: It's filled with vitamins B6, A and C, potassium, fiber and thiamin – plus folic acid (the big O helper), and vitamin E, which stimulates sex hormones in both males and females. So its benefits seem to be in that gray area between actual aphrodisiac effects and the power of suggestion. ✂

GROWING TIPS

Asparagus is relatively easy to grow in the right conditions. Plant it in average, medium, well-drained soil with a basic pH of 6.5 or higher, in full sun to part shade.

Since it takes two to three years to begin harvesting asparagus, it's best to start plants from roots, called crowns, rather than from seed (which can be tricky). This gives a jumpstart on production.

Avocado ✿ *Persea Americana*

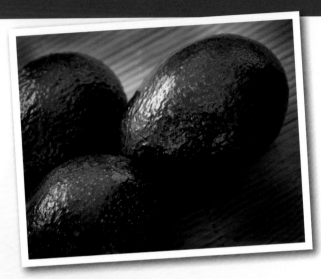

Bad news for Aztec virgins

$\mathcal{S}$EEING IS BELIEVING. AVOCADOES WERE CULTIVATED IN CENTRAL MEXICO ALMOST 10,000 years ago by the early Mayans, but Europeans didn't discover the fruit until the 16th century when Spanish conquistadores saw it under cultivation by the Aztecs. These ancient civilizations practiced their version of the Doctrine of Signatures, or the idea that an object's appearance indicated its use; thus, the testicle-like shape of the avocado showed its potent sexual powers.

A bold signature. The Aztecs dubbed the tree *āhuacatl* (pronounced ah-hoo-ah-cattle), which literately translates to "testicle"– probably due to the fruit's tendency to grow and hang in pairs. Since most of us don't live in the tropical climates needed to grow avocados, we're not likely to see them as nature intended – and thus reap the added benefit of the power of suggestion. Yet, do we intuitively know there are aphrodisiac secrets with this plant?

The avocado's aphrodisiac reputation was so widely known (and feared) by the Aztecs that

AVOCADO

Family: Lauraceae

Type: Broadleaf evergreen shrub

Color: Dark green

Harvest Period: Depending on the variety, from spring to summer

Size: 30-60 feet high; 20-30 feet wide

Soil: Deep, well-drained soil

Exposure: Full sun

Watering: Medium

pH: 6 to 6.5

Cold Hardiness Zone: 10 to 12, indoors 4 to 11

Origin: Mexico, Central America, South America

parents kept their virgin daughters indoors during the harvest of the "fertility fruit." In 1672, when King Charles II of England's personal physician encountered avocados in Jamaica, he wrote: "It nourisheth and strengtheneth the body… procuring lust exceedingly."

Lust aside, the avocado – with its lovely taste and texture – is a popular fruit commonly used in many culinary dishes. One of my favorite treats is a classic guacamole (see recipe on page 16).

Why It Works: A Closer Look

What the Mayans and Aztecs believed about the "fertility fruit" was eventually confirmed in the laboratory – at least for men. A single avocado contains 23% of the recommended daily allowance of folate (B9), and folate stimulates semen production. Also rich in zinc, B6, potassium and omega-3 fatty acids, among an impressively long list, the avocado is one of the most nutritious fruits you can eat. We know that proper nutrition is linked to health and high energy levels, opening the door for an active sex life.

GROWING TIPS

Our access to avocados is typically from a grocery store. For those of us who experience the four seasons every year, we won't be able to grow avocados, since a frost-free climate is needed. Unless… you grow it as a decorative houseplant.

In the produce section, you might notice two types of avocados – the smaller Guatemalan types, with thick, pebbly skin, and the larger Mexican types with smooth skin. The fruit ripens only after it's been picked, and until then it is actually "stored" on the tree until needed. How cool is that?

Best Guacamole from the Garden

From the kitchen of
Carolyn Binder,
Cowlick Cottage Farm

Serves 5

Our aphrodisiac friend the avocado is the main ingredient in guacamole. There are other friends from our O-list as well, including cilantro, garlic, and tomato. Guacamole is a simple summer staple (and a year-round treat with purchased fruits and vegetables from the supermarket). As Carolyn says, "Guacamole is a food for gods and gardeners. With its origins from our neighbors in Mexico, it is simple to make this an everyday food."

INGREDIENTS

¼ cup finely chopped white onion

2 tablespoons minced cilantro

3-4 jalapeño chile peppers, stemmed, seeded and finely chopped

2 cloves garlic, minced

Kosher salt, to taste

3 ripe avocados, halved, pitted, peeled, and sliced

1 tomato, cored, seeded and finely chopped

Juice of 1 lime

PREPARATION

In a large bowl or molcajete, combine onion, cilantro, peppers and garlic. Sprinkle with salt and mash with a pestle into a chunky paste.

Add avocados, tomato, and lime juice. Stir to combine, mashing the avocado as you stir. Season with salt, and serve with fresh tortilla chips or multi-grain crackers.

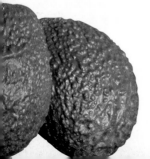

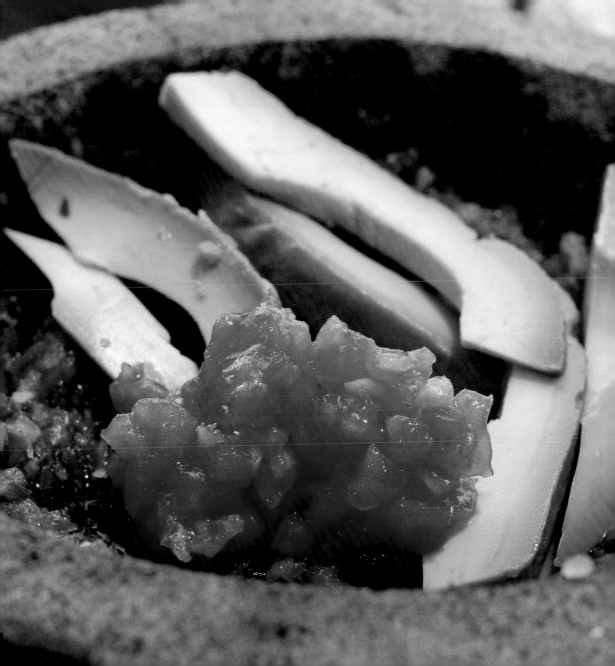

Banana ✨ *Musa acuminata*

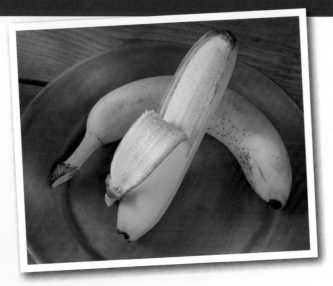

Boosts the male libido...

*B*ANANAS ARE SO COMMON IN OUR CULTURE THAT IT'S EASY TO TAKE THIS healthy fruit for granted. They're sold in grocery stores, coffee shops... even 7-Elevens. You're surely familiar with the sight of a single banana (called a finger) – and there's no getting around its amusingly phallic appearance. As other plants in this book illustrate, the human mind responds naturally to suggestive shapes.

A plant for all cultures. It seems like each generation believes they invented sex, but in truth, it's age-old, and so are the jokes associated with it. Humor aside, the shape of the banana was embraced early on in history as a fertility aid and aphrodisiac. In India, bananas were said to be a favorite of the sages, and even today, Hindus include them in offerings to the fertility gods. When a Hindu marriage is planned, the groom's family brings offerings of bananas to the family of the bride. In some Islamic traditions, it was the banana, not the apple, that was the forbidden fruit eaten in

BANANA

Family: Musaceae

Type: Herbaceous perennial

Color: Yellow

Harvest Period: Throughout the year

Size: 12 to 20 feet tall and 6 to 10 feet wide

Soil: Rich fertile soil

Exposure: Full sun

Watering: Moist

pH: 5.5 to 6.5

Cold Hardiness Zone: 10 to 11

Origin: Southeast Asia

the Garden of Eden. In Central America, the sap of the red banana tree is sipped as an aphrodisiac elixir. There must be something going on.

Why It Works: A Closer Look

So here we have a fruit with a phallic shape, and we have the human mind that can be turned on by the mere sight of objects suggestive of genitals. But let's look at this lovely fruit another way, for its measurable benefits. The importance of eating a banana is widely known, either before or after physical activity. Its nutrients, especially potassium, provide a host of positive functions for a healthy body. For men's health, many of the banana's nutrients are essential to sex hormone production, including B vitamins and potassium (for prostate health). Bananas boost the male libido because they are chock-full of chelating minerals, which help the body absorb these essential nutrients.

GROWING TIPS

The bunch of bananas that you buy in the store is most likely Musa acuminata, *a part of the* Musaceae *family. The banana originated from Asia and was introduced to the Caribbean and Central America by early Portuguese and Spanish explorers. Bananas are one of the earliest cultivated fruits, eaten by most of us on a daily basis.*

You can try to grow bananas at home, but they aren't likely to be hardy unless you live in a tropical region, and even then the tree may not fruit. Commercial bananas are grown in tropical regions where the average temperature is 80° F (27°C). So for this one, you're probably safe sticking to your local grocery store.

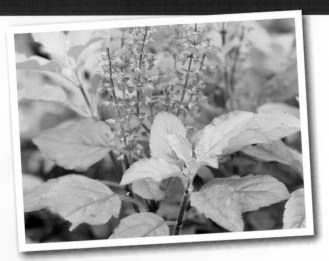

Getting action through aromatherapy

*A*NYONE WHO HAS EVER TASTED FRESH BASIL KNOWS THE DISTINCTIVE FLAVOR of this herb. Basil, combined with garlic, olive oil and pine nuts, as well as Parmesan cheese and a dash of salt, melds into an infusion with endless applications for pastas, soups, and spreads. As a food, basil adds a decadent flavor, but did you know basil is also a symbol of love?

Four thousand years ago, in Malaysia, Iran and Egypt, basil was used as a love token, and laid at the gravesite of loved ones. In Hindu belief, holy basil symbolizes love.

Basil is also associated with the Haitian love goddess, Erzulie Fréda. Erzulie wore three wedding rings, one for each husband. Basil water placed on her altar will draw her to your prayers for love.

Rub basil... where? The basil most of us grow is sweet basil, *Ocimum basilicum* (a mood changer in its own right), but the basil that made aphrodisiac history is holy basil,

HOLY BASIL

Featured Plant: Holy basil, *Ocimum tenuiflorum*

Family: Lamiaceae, mint family

Color: Green with pink, white, or near-white flower

Harvest Period: June to frost. Keep from going to flower; pinched back

Type: Tender perennial herb, treated as an annual

Size: 2 to 3 feet high and wide

Soil: Moderately rich, well-drained soil

Exposure: Full sun

Watering: Moist; do not let the soil dry out.

pH: 6.4

Cold Hardiness Zone: 10 to 11; grown as an annual in warm climates

Origin: Tropical India, Asia, and Africa

Ocimum tenuiflorum (syn. *O. sanctum*), also known as tulsi. In ancient times, women would rub dry basil powder on their bodies to become more sexually attractive. In Italy today, sweet basil is the symbol of love and is called *"bacia-nicola,"* or "kiss me Nicholas." Placed on the windowsill, it signals for a lover.

Why It Works: A Closer Look

Basil is a wonderful all-purpose aphrodisiac getting action through aromatherapy – it's the smell of basil that drives us wild. This herb has been known to stimulate the sex drive and induce a general sense of well being for the mind and body. And according to the International Journal of Ayurveda Research, holy basil increases testosterone levels in men.

GROWING TIPS

All basil is easy to grow, but it needs warm weather to thrive. Very frost sensitive, it will not tolerate a dip into cold nighttime temperatures.

Sow seeds in full sun, buried a half-inch deep, two to three inches apart. Once seedlings appear, thin to one foot apart. Basil is also readily available as a bedding plant from your local garden center. Set nursery plants 10 to 12 inches apart. Basil also does very well as a container plant; just keep it well watered.

Holy and sweet basil are grown as a summer annual, reaching two to three feet high. Each time you pinch it back for dinner or dessert, you help maintain the size. Keep the flowers pinched off to encourage bushiness and leaf production – though the flowers are tasty too.

Basil Pesto

From the kitchen of
Carolyn Binder,
Cowlick Cottage Farm

Yield: about 1 cup

Basil pesto is one way that it's OK to be "spread thin" – or, you can be lavish with it. A flavorful condiment chock-full of contentment, basil pesto is an aphrodisiac spread where even a little dab will do ya.

INGREDIENTS

2 cups fresh basil leaves (packed)
1/3 cup pine nuts
3 medium sized garlic cloves, minced
1/2 cup extra virgin olive oil (EVOO)
1/2 cup freshly grated Parmesan-Reggiano
Salt and pepper, to taste

PREPARATION

In a food processor, combine basil with pine nuts. Pulse a few times.
Add garlic and pulse some more.

While hand stirring, slowly add the EVOO.

Add the grated cheese and pulse one more time.
Add salt and pepper to taste.

Serve at room temperature. It makes a sensual dipping sauce for breads or baguette slices, or you can pour it over pasta for a light and refreshing entree.

Pesto can be refrigerated. It also freezes well. Divide the batch (or double batch) into sandwich size baggies. The more you make, the better your winter feasting will be.

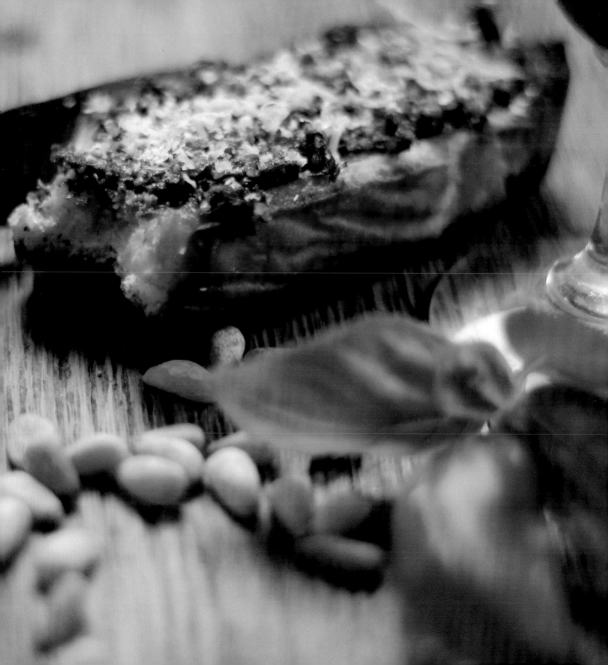

Cardamom   ❧ *Elettaria cardamomum*

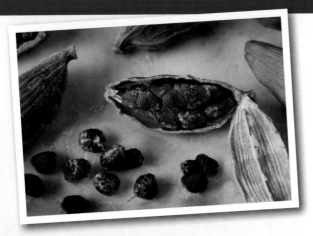

One whiff is all you need

ON MANY MIDDLE EASTERN COUNTRIES, THE DAYBREAK AIR IS SCENTED WITH AN enticing blend of coffee and seed. This morning ritual combines the bitterness of a good strong coffee bean with the sweet, pungent flavor of the cardamom seed.

For more than 3,000 years in India, Ayurvedic medicine has used cardamom to treat a myriad of maladies to reduce pain, lift the spirits and restore vitality, with particular attention to the releasing of nervous tension – and as an aphrodisiac. With its sweet, fresh, uplifting aroma, cardamom can banish worries with a single whiff.

Irresistible. We find cardamom mentioned as an aphrodisiac in that collection of magical tales, *The Arabian Nights*. Cardamom has a long history as an ingredient in a number of ancient love spells. If you believe the way to a man's heart is through his stomach, than the Greeks perfected the ideal love potion with baklava.

Today, cardamom is used in a variety of ways, from traditional curry powders to flavoring confectioneries and liqueurs – and even chewing gum (in Mexico and Guatemala). Scandinavians use more cardamom than anyone else in the Western Hemisphere, consuming almost half

CARDAMOM

Family: Zingiberaceae

Type: Tender perennial, tropical

Color: Green foliage with white (or near white) blooms

Harvest Period: Spring

Size: 12 feet tall

Soil: Rich loamy

Exposure: Partial to Full Shade

Watering: Moist

pH: 5.1 to 6.5

Cold Hardiness Zone: Zone 10 to 12, above freezing, constant temperature around 72° F/ 22°C is best.

Origin: India

of the world's supply for baking, flavoring meatballs, pickled herring, and in aquavit, a spirit that has been produced in Scandinavia since the 15th century.

The aroma of cardamom is so alluring (some would say intoxicating), it's often used in perfumery. The seeds can be made into sachets for the linen drawer. Fresh linens scented with cardamom could be the prelude to an "ancient evening" of delights.

Why It Works: A Closer Look

Traditionally, cardamom is considered a powerful aphrodisiac with the ability to treat impotence. It has, however, been suggested that cardamom's reputation springs from its aroma and its warming effects when drunk as a tea. What we can say is that cardamom is warming and pungent – and high in cineole, which can increase blood flow.

Macerate cardamom pods in hot water to make a classic Indian tea, or chai, or add to your favorite stir-fried dishes. ✂

GROWING TIPS

Cardamom is the dried, unripened fruit of the tropical perennial plant, Elettaria cardamomum. Also known as green cardamom, this spice is a member of the ginger family, Zingiberaceae. The fruit is picked when unripe, then dried. The dried spice comes in pods that can ground for use as needed.

Cardamom will flower and fruit only in tropical regions; in cooler climates, cardamom will make an attractive foliage plant. Plant in a shady, moist border or bed.

Carrot 🌿 *Daucus carota* var. *sativus*

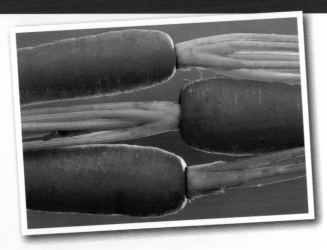

The ancient love charm

*S*ERIOUSLY? ALL IT TAKES FOR A MAN'S AROUSAL IS THE SIGHT OF A CARROT?! Maybe they should be used more for decorations around the house – ornaments on the Christmas tree, for a pull cord from the ceiling fan light, and sitting in a clear vase on top of the television. Women should start a new tradition of sending your man a bouquet of carrots for no special reason other than you want to love him (and for him to love on you, but he doesn't have to know that!).

Archaeological evidence of the wild carrot dates back to Mesolithic times – 10,000 years ago – with indications that the gathered seeds were used for medicinal purposes.

The phallus-shaped carrot (albeit rather pointy) has been associated with aphrodisiac stimulation since ancient times. Middle Eastern royalty used this vegetable in stimulation and to aid in seduction.

The Greeks referred to the carrot as a philtron, meaning a love potion or love charm (from *philos*, meaning loving). Dioscorides, the 1st century A.D. physician and botanist, wrote that

CARROT

Family: Apiaceae

Type: Biennial vegetable, considered an annual if not grown for the seed

Color: Orange

Harvest Period: Spring

Size: 0.25 to 3 feet high and wide

Soil: Deep, loose and well-drained

Exposure: Full sun

Watering: Medium

pH: 6.0 to 6.8

Cold Hardiness Zone: 2 to 11

Origin: Afghanistan

the root, among its many medicinal benefits, was an aphrodisiac. The Romans also believed in the carrot's aphrodisiac attributes. Carrots were common in a Roman garden, where the root and seed were thought to increase the libido.

The color of love. The carrots of these earlier times were the color purple, with mutated versions occasionally popping up, including yellow and white, instead of our familiar sunset-glow orange. That didn't happen until the 17th century, when Dutch

growers took mutant strains of the purple carrot and gradually developed them into a sweet, plump, orange variety. They were further cultivated for a sweeter taste, leading up to the veggie we serve today.

Why It Works: A Closer Look

Carrots are rich in beta-carotene and vitamin A. Quite nutritious and good for the eyes and all that, but when it comes right down to it, the carrot's aphrodisiac success must be attributed to its shape. Yes, we are simple creatures. ✄

GROWING TIPS

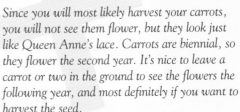

Today's carrots were cultivated from the wild carrot Daucus carota var. carota, which is the weedy Queen Anne's lace native to Europe and Asia, and has naturalized in North American fields and roadsides.

Since you will most likely harvest your carrots, you will not see them flower, but they look just like Queen Anne's lace. Carrots are biennial, so they flower the second year. It's nice to leave a carrot or two in the ground to see the flowers the following year, and most definitely if you want to harvest the seed.

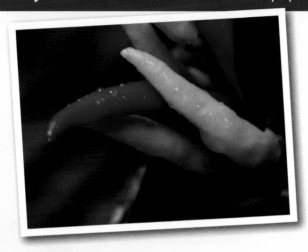

Rev things up for hot fun!

ℋAVE YOU SEEN THE MOVIE CHOCOLAT? I WAS MESMERIZED BY IT. BUT IT wasn't the late 1950s French village setting (for which I'm always a sucker), the continued appeal of the quirky Johnny Depp, or even the beautiful Juliette Binoche that kept my attention; I was preoccupied with wondering what the heroine, Vianne Rocher, was putting in that chocolate! Whatever it was, it cured everyone who consumed her delectables. Sure, they may have killed Judy Dench's character, but at least she died happy.

It's all about the heat. Vianne's secret was the red-hot chili pepper, also known as cayenne. Cayenne *(Capsicum annuum)* is not actually a pepper at all, but a berry, making it a member of the genus Capsicum.

There is evidence that cayenne pepper was in use in Central and South America as early as 7,000 B.C., but the combination of cayenne and chocolate was discovered later, in the ancient Aztec culture, where the royalty in particular enjoyed a little heat with their treat.

CAYENNE

Family: Solanaceae

Type: Perennial small shrub, grown as an annual

Color: Showy, edible fruit

Harvest Period: Seasonal, summer

Size: 1 to 4 feet high and 1 to 2 feet wide

Soil: Moist, well-drained

Exposure: Full sun

Watering: Medium, tolerates drought

pH: 5.5 to 7.5

Cold Hardiness Zone: Grown as an annual

Origin: Tropical North and South America

Christopher Columbus introduced cayenne to Europe and wrote about its medicinal effects in 1494. Cayenne became so popular that in 1767 young Thomas Jefferson planted it at his birthplace home at Shadwell. I'm not sure Jefferson was aware of cayenne's amorous properties, but nonetheless he explored growing this perky, heat-enhancing berry with its peppers erect toward the sky.

Why It Works: A Closer Look

There is little to support that cayenne has any properties in large enough quantities to make it a medically sought-after aphrodisiac, but its reputation as one still persists. Why? It's actually appreciated as a local stimulant that can rev things up for hot fun in the summertime.

Cayenne is considered a warming herb because its effects mimic our body's sexual stimulation responses. The increased heart rate and dilated blood vessels improve blood flow throughout the body, particularly to the major organs. Nothing like some capsicum in your diet to get a little heat in the loins! ✄

GROWING TIPS

Cayenne peppers are an easy-to-grow annual that prefer moist, organically rich, well-drained soils. They grow well in containers. Plant out in your garden bed or container in full sun after the threat of your last spring frost date. Depending on your growing season, start seeds inside or buy seedlings from your local garden center.

The plant itself can be pinched back to promote a more bushy form, and cayenne peppers can be eaten in a color-state from green to red.

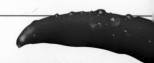

Hot Cocoa, Vianne Style

Makes 2 mugs

Hot cocoa on a cold winter's day is a welcome treat. For me, it often conjures up the childhood memories of wearing wet mittens, wrapped around the warm mug, as I wait to take the first sip. But this isn't your mamma's hot chocolate. There is a kick to it, worthy of a more grown-up taste.

INGREDIENTS

16 ounces whole milk

2 tablespoons double chocolate cocoa

6 tablespoons Dutch processed cocoa powder

½ teaspoon ground cinnamon

¼ teaspoon ground cayenne pepper

¼ teaspoon ground nutmeg

PREPARATION

In a small saucepan, heat the milk to just before it boils.

Add the double chocolate cocoa, Dutch processed cocoa powder, and spices. Mix until blended.

Serve in a beautiful mugs and garnish with a dollop of whipped cream.

For even more of a kick to your taste buds, try substituting a chili pepper for the cayenne!

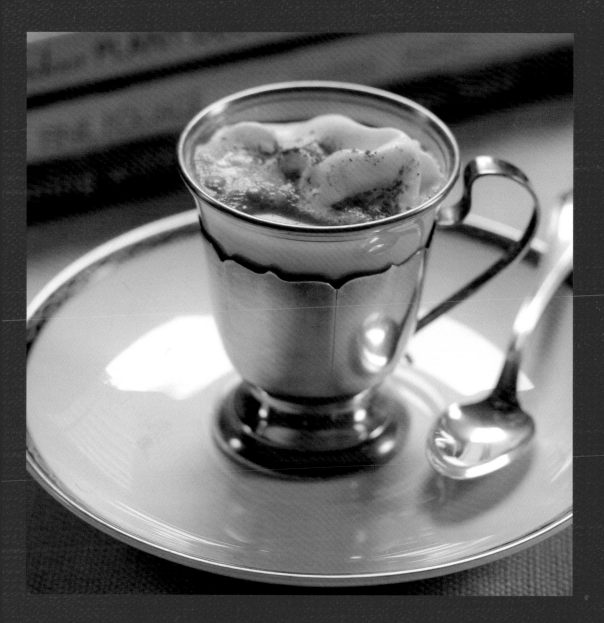

Casanova's secret weapon

ℭELERY IS NOT EXACTLY MY FIRST, SECOND, OR 50TH FAVORITE SNACK FOOD. It's not that I don't like it, and when smeared with peanut butter, it's good; but I can just eat the peanut butter right off the spoon. Honestly, the spoon tastes about the same as celery, so why bother? But heed me: once you learn about the benefits of this plant, your toes will perk up with interest.

I can see how its reputation as an aphrodisiac might come from the shape of the individual stalks, but that takes some imagination. Visual stimimulus or not, some recent studies suggest celery will indeed enhance your libido.

A sexy *and* wholesome plant? Long associated with male potency and vigor, sexuality, mental clarity, and fertility, celery has been cultivated for over 3,000 years (a garland woven with celery was found in an early Egyptian tomb). The ancient Greeks called it *selinon*, regarding it as a holy plant. Homer mentioned its health benefits in his *Odyssey*, and in the Greek

Celery

Family: Apiaceae (or Umbelliferae), carrot family

Color: Light green leaf stalks

Harvest Period: Spring seasonal

Type: Biennial vegetable

Size: 10 inches high and 6 inches wide

Soil: Rich soil, high in organic matter

Exposure: Full sun

Watering: Moist

pH: 6 to 6.5

Cold Hardiness Zone: Although it is a cool-season crop, exposure of juvenile plants to temperatures below 40 to 50°F for more than 5 to 10 days can cause premature bolting, ruining the crop.

Origin: Native to Europe and the Mediterranean region, and cultivated there for over 3,000 years

Nemean Games, celery leaves were worn as garlands by the victors. But the Romans preferred eating celery over using it ceremonially. However, that famous Italian lover Casanova was known to eat celery regularly to stimulate his libido. In France, the 18th century food writer Grimod de la Reyniere cautioned his readers about celery: "It is enough to stress that it is not in any way a salad for bachelors." Wink wink.

Why It Works: A Closer Look

Celery is packed with an organic chemical called phthalide. This compound is capable of dilating blood vessels, improving circulation, having an impact on the ability to have and maintain an erection. But also, celery may enhance the synthesis of the steroid androstenone, which is released in men's perspiration as a pheromone, and has been known to act as a sexual attractant. Deep breaths, ladies... ✄

GROWING TIPS

Celery is considered a cut-and-come-again vegetable. If celery is harvested on a regular basis, it will send up new stalks.

This biennial plant is best grown in cool seasons or climates and moist, well-drained soil. Celery tolerates shade, which makes it a great choice for gardens with too little sun. It's not the easiest plant to grow, but celery is readily available at the grocery store.

Celery with a Side of Bloody Mary

From the kitchen of
Carolyn Binder,
Cowlick Cottage Farm

A Cocktail for 2

The practice of using celery to garnish a Bloody Mary originated in the 1960s at Chicago's Ambassador East Hotel. A patron was served a Bloody Mary without a swizzle stick. The story goes that he reached over and grabbed a stalk of celery from the relish tray to stir his drink. He loved the addition and the rest is history.

You can make your Celery with a Side of Bloody Mary cocktail as spicy or mild as you like, but remember that the capsicum from the cayenne pepper (also found in hot sauce) increases your amorous potential (see page 28).

INGREDIENTS

8 ounces tomato juice
1½ ounce vodka
1½ ounce lemon juice
Dash of Worcestershire sauce, to taste
Pinch of celery salt
Pinch of fresh ground pepper
Hot pepper sauce, to taste
Celery stalk, for garnish

PREPARATION

Mix the liquid ingredients in a pitcher.
Add seasonings to taste.

Stir, and pour into highball glasses
over ice.

Garnish with celery stalks and serve.

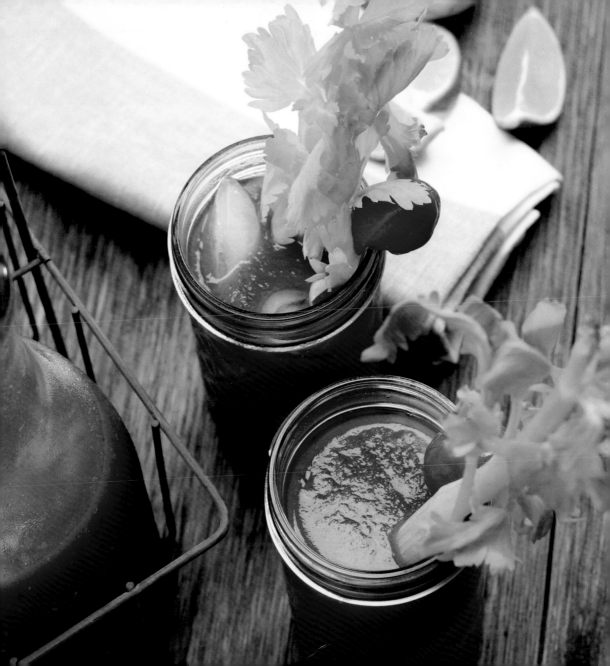

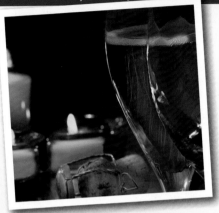

Bubbles galore
and a whole
lot more

℘OP. FIZZLE. GIGGLE. IT'S THE SEQUENCE THAT HAPPENS WHEN CHAMPAGNE shares your evening's plans. The excitement typically begins when some special occasion warrants popping the cork of a champagne bottle.

Champagne was Marilyn Monroe's favorite drink; what glamorous red-carpet star doesn't like having a stem of delicate bubbles? Even the curvy champagne glass is sensual. Champagne wasn't always viewed as mankind's sexiest drink, though.

A happy mistake. During the Middle Ages in northern France, still wine was the way to go, but cold winters there – particularly in the area of Champagne – caused alcohol's fermentation process to stop prematurely. When the weather warmed again, sugar and carbon dioxide in the wine bottle would cause bubbling to occur. Though you might be happy about those bubbles in what we know today as sparkling wine, the French in the 17th century were none too pleased.

While the French Benedictine monks were trying to still the unruly bubbles, the English were becoming fond of the strange brew. Eventually, sparkling wine became popular world-

CHAMPAGNE GRAPES

Family: Vitaceae

Type: Deciduous, edible vine

Color: Good fall color, small, dark purple grapes

Harvest Period: Fall

Size: 15 - 20 feet high and 8 feet wide

Soil: Well-drained, fertile

Exposure: Full sun

Watering: Medium

pH: 6.5 to 7

Cold Hardiness Zone: 7 to 10

Origin: Western Asia

---

wide, and the *méthode champenoise* – the process of adding yeast and sugar to base wine – was created.

Sidenote: In 1846, Pierre-Nicolas-Marie Perrier-Jouët brewed champagne without sugar. His "brutal"-flavored drink took a while to catch on, but then "extra dry" brut became popular as well. Out with the old, in with the new!

Why It Works: A Closer Look

Like all alcohol, champagne loosens inhibition, particularly when sipped in moderation. This bubbly drink also hits the blood stream more quickly than still wine, filling the body with warm desire. Its aphrodisiac allure is not with the effervescence alone, however. Dr. Max Lake, an Australian surgeon, vintner and researcher, suggests the scent of champagne mimics the delicate aromas of the female pheromones.

Champagne also contains trace minerals of magnesium, potassium and zinc – all essential for both male and female sex hormone production. ✀

GROWING TIPS

Most champagne is a blend of up to three grape varieties: Pinot noir, Chardonnay and Pinot Meunier. Realistically, you won't be bottling your own bubbly drink, so my featured plant isn't one or all of those. Instead, it is the fruit of a variety called 'Black Corinth', commonly referred to as "champagne grapes" because its tiny grapes resemble the bubbles in our titular drink. This variety is named for the Greek city where they were grown more than 2,000 years ago.

To enjoy their sweet flavor and pleasant crunch in all climate zones, you'll do best to buy them at your grocer's.

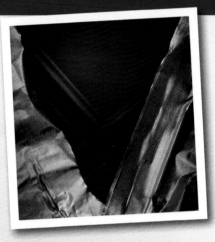

Feels a lot like being in love...

*N*OTHING SAYS LOVE LIKE CHOCOLATE – YOU LOVE THE TASTE, YOU LOVE THE gift, you love the love that comes within a heart-shaped box of sweets.

The cacao bean genus Theobroma originated millions of years ago in what we know as South America. Fast forward over a thousand millennia, and we have evidence that the Mayans domesticated cacao and that it was being drunk by traders as early as 400 B.C. It was given the name "Food of the Gods." The later Aztec culture, which dominated in Mesoamerica from the 14th century to the Spanish Conquest, placed much emphasis on the virtue of cacao.

The first outsider to drink chocolate was Christopher Columbus, when he reached Nicaragua in 1502. The chocolate drink was not what we think of today, but rather a bitter, spicy, pure dark chocolate refreshment called *xocoatl*, but it was clear the precursor of the modern winter delight we call hot chocolate. Once cacao was introduced to Spain in 1528, sugar was added, making it a popular drink in the Spanish royal courts.

Montezuma's rendezvous. It is thought that the Aztecs were the first to draw a link between the cocoa bean and sexual desire. The story goes that the Aztec ruler Montezuma

CHOCOLATE

Family: Malvaceae

Type: Broadleaf evergreen

Color: Showy pink flowers, edible fruit

Harvest Period: Cacao is an interesting plant in that it flowers and fruits at the same time, so harvesting is done almost year round.

Size: 20 to 30 feet high and wide

Soil: A wide range of soil types

Exposure: Full sun to part shade

Watering: Medium

pH: 5 to 7.5

Cold Hardiness Zone: 11

Origin: Central and South America, to the east of the Andes.

A Milan study with women subjects linked the consumption of chocolate and the feeling of sexual fulfillment. Those who ate chocolate daily reported a higher degree of sexual satisfaction – even from women who normally had a lower libido.

Other studies attribute chocolate's aphrodisiac qualities to three chemicals that are thought of as "the love drugs": phenylethylamine (PEA), tryptophan, and anandamide (AEA), each with the ability to stimulate the pleasure centers. Cacao also contains flavonoids, which help promote blood vessel health, meaning blood easily flows throughout the body.

One thing we can say with confidence: it does make us feel good all over – much like being in love.

called it "the divine drink" and consumed 50 goblets of cacao daily for strength. Did he also mean sexual strength?

Why It Works: A Closer Look

It's debated if chocolate is indeed an aphrodisiac, but studies suggest it has merit. Research reveals cacao as a mood-lifter, which leads to the feeling of excitement, as well as increasing one's level of energy, and thus receptivity to desire.

GROWING TIPS

Cacao, Theobroma cacao, is a member of the Malvaceae family along with cotton and hibiscus. Cacao's natural habitat is the lower story of the evergreen rainforest. Since we are not likely to have those climatic conditions in our own back gardens, I encourage you to purchase fair-trade chocolate and stimulate yourself with one square at a time.

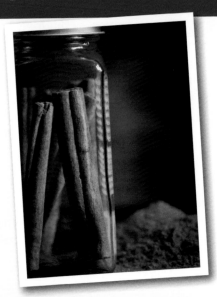

Not just for pumpkin pie...

*W*HAT WOULD OUR HOLIDAY SEASONS BE LIKE WITHOUT CINNAMON? FROM flavoring cider during a crisp fall Halloween evening to pumpkin and apple pies for our Thanksgiving feast, cinnamon is found in nearly every American home. Three thousand years ago, it also spiced up the bedchamber.

A warm and romantic scent. In Proverbs 7 of the Old Testament, the biblical lover says, "I have perfumed my bed with myrrh, aloes and cinnamon. Come, let us take our fill of love till morning." Cinnamon is also mentioned in the Song of Solomon, where the beloved's garments smell of "Spikenard and saffron; calamus and cinnamon..." Later, in Rome, the word cinnamon was a term of affection, like "darling." Scent and spice were clearly the language of love from way back.

Cinnamon

Family: Lauracea

Type: Tropical broadleaf evergreen

Color: Cinnamon brown

Color: During rainy season

Size: 25 to 50 Feet tall and 30 to 75 feet wide

Soil: Tolerant of a wide range of soils.

Exposure: Full sun to part shade

Watering: Wet climate

pH: 6.2 and below

Cold Hardiness Zone: Tropical 10 to 15; no extremes of heat and cold

Origin: Ceylon (today's Sri Lanka)

Each part of the cinnamon tree – leaves, flower buds and bark – is used to make the spice and essential oils, each yielding a different product. The part we know best is from the tree bark, which is first stripped down to the brown inner layer, then allowed to dry, turning into those familiar stick-like quills. This part yields the highest of the essential oil cinnamaldehyde. Served in hot drinks and pies and all manner of confections, cinnamon has a "something special" that many of us crave without knowing why.

Why It Works: A Closer Look

Other than the obvious emotional appeal of its aromatic oils, there isn't much science to support cinnamon as an aphrodisiac. However, cinnamon bark is considered a warming agent, producing heat in the body and increasing circulation in the pelvic region (and all the good that comes from that!).

But wait: it has recently been found that men are particularly affected by the scent of cinnamon, which can cause arousal with a single inhalation. You can test the theory with the recipe on the next page. ✄

GROWING TIPS

Cinnamon, Cinnamomum verum (syn. Cinnamomum zeylandicum), is a slow-growing, tropical broadleaf evergreen tree of the Lauracea family of plants, along with avocado, bay laurel and camphor. Sadly, most of us will not be able to grow a cinnamon tree outside in our home gardens, since it requires a warm, wet, tropical climate, with no extremes of hot or cold. Cinnamon trees will tolerate bright shade, though, and can be grown as a houseplant. The good news: cinnamon sticks and ground cinnamon are widely available in the spice section of our local grocery store. Let's make some buns, babe!

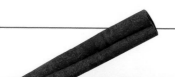

Pumpkin Pie Tarts

Yield: 36 tarts

This would be a sensual treat even if you didn't know it contained four aphrodisiac spices. Enjoy!

INGREDIENTS

2 eggs, lightly beaten

1 14-ounce can pumpkin

1 cup brown sugar, packed

1 teaspoon cinnamon

½ teaspoon nutmeg

½ teaspoon ginger paste

¼ teaspoon clove

½ teaspoon salt

¾ cup evaporated milk

36 frozen tart shells (2-inch size)

PREPARATION

Preheat over to 425 °F.

In a large bowl, combine all ingredients gently with a spatula.

Spoon batter into tart shells and place onto an ungreased cookie sheet.

Bake for 15 minutes. Then reduce heat to 350°F and bake for another 30 minutes.

Remove immediately from cookie sheet onto cooling racks.

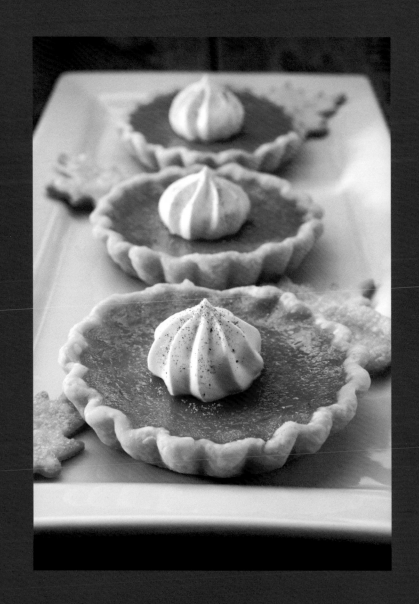

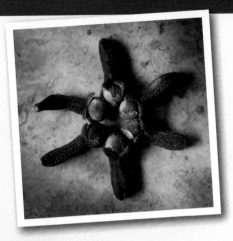

A stimulating flower part

CLOVES WERE THE FIRST SPICE TO BE TRADED, WITH EVIDENCE OF CLOVES found in vessels dating as far back as 1,721 B.C. The ancient Romans treasured cloves. In China's Han Dynasty (3rd century B.C. to 3rd century A.D.) cloves were used for cooking and in medicine; and if you had an audience with the emperor, you were instructed to chew cloves to freshen your breath. It was known to be an aphrodisiac as well – its oil and its scent.

There is now some science behind this sexually stimulating flower part, but even absent that, the shape is so sensual, your mind would have eventually gone there. I wonder if that is why my mother so lovingly took her time inserting cloves into the holiday ham?

How did clove get its name? Cloves resemble small nails (the word is derived from the Latin, *clavus*, meaning nail). Also, the Spanish word for clove is *clavo*, meaning nail. It's hard not to notice the phallic shape. So it's no wonder that a distasteful term for a sexual conquest is to *nail her*. To those boys who say that, read more and learn that plants are about love, not conquest.

CLOVES

Family: Myrtaceae

Type: Evergreen tree

Color: Rich brown; cloves are the aromatic dried flower buds of the tree.

Harvest Period: Spring and winter. Trees only begin producing flowers after about 20 years. Very slow growing, but clove trees live a long time.

Soil: Rich loamy

Exposure: Full sun to partial shade

Watering: Moist

pH: 6.0 to 7.5

Cold Hardiness Zone: Tropical zones 10 - 11

Origin: Indonesia

Equal opportunity. Cloves alleviate a toothache by anesthetizing the nerve. Well, the Chinese figured out that if the male applied clove oil to his, um, penis, then it would help with premature ejaculation. The libido of both sexes, however, can be stimulated by drinking a concoction of cloves, cinnamon and ginger – with some sherry to help things along.

Why It Works: A Closer Look

Cloves contain eugenol, an effective local anesthetic; its aromatic fragrance is thought to enhance sexual feelings. Clove oil also naturally heats up the body to put you in the mood. If you believe the Swiss mice from a 2003 study, clove extracts did improve their sexual performance. (I can see them after the study, standing around smoking a clove cigarette.)

The other big news comes from our old friend, the Doctrine of Signatures. This food resembles a penis, so it must help the penis, right? That's how they think, anyway. As such, shape puts cloves on the list of aphrodisiacs. ✄

GROWING TIPS

Syzygium aromaticum (syn. Eugenia caryophyllata) is commonly known as clove. Cloves come from the Myrtaceae family native to the North Moluccas, the Spice Islands of Indonesia and India. They are the immature unopened flower buds of this tropical tree.

Clove trees are very particular about where they grow, but they can make a nice houseplant. Seeds can be purchased online and should be started with a good organic soil mix.

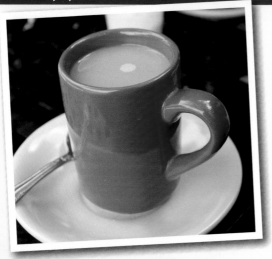

Perk up your morning... in more ways than one

ᖴORGET DOGS AS MAN'S BEST FRIEND – THE FINEST RELATIONSHIP I'VE EVER witnessed was between a man and his coffee. Each morning, my dad woke up extra early just to be alone with his cup of joe – exactly two cups. As an early riser myself, I would often catch him at the tail end of his morning love affair. I dreamed of having the same kind of relationship with coffee as my dad. Now, I rise an hour before the rest of my family to share my morning with joe – exactly two cups, just like Dad, and I'm ready to start my day.

Feelin' a little frisky. According to legend, the Ethiopian goatherd Kaldi noticed his goats were acting particularly feisty after nibbling on the leaves of a certain tree. Kaldi tried some of the plant himself and was amazed at its perky effects. Before long, mankind began cultivating coffee trees and making that bitter brew enjoyed everywhere.

From its origins in Ethiopia, Sudan, and Kenya in the 13th century, the coffee tree spread quickly to the Egyptians and Turks, through Europe, before landing with a bang in the

COFFEE

Family: Rubiaceae

Type: Broadleaf evergreen

Color: White flowers, green turning red, and blue/black drupes

Harvest Period: Once a year when the coffee cherries ripen

Size: 6 to 15 feet high and wide

Soil: Good drainage is essential; soil textures lighter than clays

Exposure: Part shade

Watering: Medium

pH: 5.2 to 6.2

Cold Hardiness Zone: 10 to 11

Origin: Ethiopia, Sudan, Kenya

Americas. In fact, Seattle was home to that coffee industry giant, Starbucks.

Why It Works: A Closer Look

While considered an aphrodisiac in many traditions, there is little scientific proof that it actually affects the libido. Despite this, coffee is still thought to stimulate sexual desire and improve male potency. According to Michael and Ellen Albertson's book *Temptations*, studies show that coffee drinkers have sex more frequently than non-coffee drinkers.

A 2011 study from the University of Vienna revealed that coffee stimulates the body by triggering the release of dopamine, the neurotransmitter associated with the pleasure system of the brain. This could account for the increased libido, as a stimulated body might be mistaken for sexual arousal.

Others argue that the caffeine in coffee increases blood flow by stimulating the heart and the body's adrenaline levels. So maybe our favorite bitter brew does have a special kick... ✁

GROWING TIPS

The coffee tree, Coffea arabica, is a member of the Rubiaceae family of flowering plants in a clan called the coffee family. Grown outdoors, the coffee tree needs a warm, frost-free climate, but Coffea arabica also makes a nice indoor plant if grown in a sunny window and taken outside on the deck or patio during the summer months.

The coffee beans are actually seeds of the tree's berries. The berries are handpicked when ripe, then de-pulped and dried in the sun before roasting.

Coriander (Cilantro) ❧ *Coriandrum sativum*

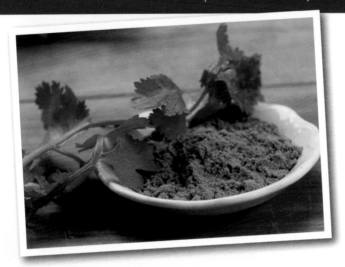

To sweeten and spice your nights

CORIANDER IS AN IMPORTANT FLAVORING IN MANY OF THE WORLD'S CUISINES. It can trace its roots back over 7,000 years, making it one of the world's oldest known spices, with archaeological evidence dating back to the Neolithic period in Israel.

It was cultivated in ancient Egypt and mentioned in the Old Testament (Exodus 16:3): "… and it [manna] was like coriander seed, white; and the taste of it was like wafers made with honey." But coriander became really famous when promoted as an aphrodisiac in *The Arabian Nights*, with a tale of a merchant who had been childless for 40 years and was cured after he drank a mixture containing coriander. The Chinese traditionally used the herb in love potions, believing it stimulated arousal and bestowed immortality.

In the Middle Ages, a popular drink served at weddings to increase the libido was called Hippocras – a blend of coriander, cardamom, clove, ginger and cinnamon, mixed with red wine

CORIANDER

Family: Apiaceae

Type: Coriander, cilantro seed

Color: Limey green

Harvest Period: End of summer

Size: 1.5 to 2 feet high and 1 to 1.5 feet wide

Soil: Loamy and well-drained

Exposure: Full sun, part shade

Watering: Medium

pH: 4.8 to 8

Cold Hardiness Zone: 2 to 11, annual grown after frost

Origin: Europe and western Mediterranean

(see recipe on page 132). Hippocras was brought to Europe from the Crusades. and then found popularity in the Americas.

Oh, that scent! Cilantro has a scent that people either love or hate. Some consider it extremely pleasant, but others are repulsed by it. There is some evidence that suggests a genetic component to these taste responses.

Why It Works: A Closer Look

Coriander is rich in vitamins, minerals and phytonutrients (it has phyto-estrogen, which helps with hormonal balance). It is also a blood purifier and digestive aid. Besides the obvious health and flavor benefits, I'm afraid we're left with only lore to support coriander as a true aphrodisiac. Perhaps it remains an aphrodisiac for many cultures because if you are in good health, you'll feel inspired to spend an evening of love. ✄

GROWING TIPS

Coriander is the seed from the Coriandrum sativum, *commonly known as cilantro. A member of the Apiaceae family, coriander is easy to grow in average, well-drained soils. Cilantro grows best in areas with cool, dry summers.*

Seeds can be sown directly into the soil or grown in containers. Plants will grow rapidly and will bolt (go to seed) when the weather gets too hot. Let the plant go to flower, then harvest the seeds. Seeds are ready to harvest in 90 days after planting.

The mature seeds have a pleasant sweet-spicy aroma and are used in flavoring foods anywhere from savory to sweet: sauces, sausages, stews, as well as chutneys, pies and cakes.

Cucumber ❧ *Cucumis sativus*

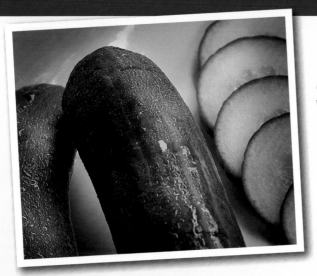

Sexual stamina in vegetable form

*H*AVE YOU EVER KICKED BACK FROM A ROUGH DAY AND SOUGHT RELIEF WITH cool, thin slices of cucumber resting on your eyelids, just like in those fancy resorts and Hollywood movies? Keeping cool as a cucumber may not be its only benefit to man- or womankind.

A well-traveled fruit. Cucumber is believed to have been cultivated throughout the Indian subcontinent for at least 3,000 years, where it has been used to temper the hot effects of spicy food, and for its many healing properties (including as a digestive aid and an anti-inflammatory). From there, it was introduced to North Africa, Greece and Rome. In 1st century Rome, the naturalist Pliny wrote of a greenhouse-type system that Emperor Tiberius had built so that he could enjoy the delicacy on his table year-round. Soon, the cucumber was a staple all over Europe and around into China. The cucumber didn't show up in North America until Christopher Columbus brought it to Haiti in 1494.

CUCUMBER

Family: Cucurbitaceae, along with squash and gourds

Type: Annual vegetable vine

Color: Green

Harvest Period: Summer, seasonal bloomer

Size: 3 to 8 feet high and wide

Soil: Rich organic, well-drained soil

Exposure: Full sun

Watering: Medium

pH: 5.5 - 7

Cold Hardiness Zone: 2 to 11

Origin: East Indies

Popular and tasty, yes, but that doesn't make it a "hot" item for our purposes. Read on.

Why It Works: A Closer Look

To the casual observer, you might think the cucumber's aphrodisiac benefits rely only on its profile (a natural for the Doctrine of Signatures). While it is certainly phallic in appearance, there are some studies to suggest its aphrodisiac attributes aren't based on looks alone. One study, by Dr. Alan Hirsch,

found that the scent of cucumbers, in combination with black licorice, caused arousal in women. Men, take note, because certain scents can drive women wild, and it's not whatever stuff is in that bottle with a ship on it.

In certain corners of the alternative healthcare world, cucumbers have been linked to sexual stamina and have even been called the organic Viagra. Nutritionally, cucumbers are rich in potassium, which helps with hypertension (which can contribute to erectile dysfunction). It also provides a slew of other nutrients essential to maintaining sexual health. ✂

GROWING TIPS

Cucumbers are easily grown in loose, slightly acidic (pH 5.5 to 7), organically rich, and well-drained soil. Plant in full sun and give a lot of space for common vining varieties to sprawl. Climbing cucumbers can also be trellised or trained in cages to bring off the ground; this is particularly helpful in home gardens with limited space. Keep well watered; consistent and even moisture is essential.

There are several varieties to choose from, depending on whether you favor short or long fruit and if you want a vine or a bush (such as the Burpless Bush Hybrid).

Tomato, Broccoli, Cucumber & Cilantro Salad

From the kitchen of
Shawna Coronado

Makes 2-plus cups

This aphrodisiac salad promises to delight more than a few of your senses and trigger the release of those feel-good endorphins. It's mostly about the cucumber, tomato and cilantro, of course, but the broccoli and Italian dressing are a bonus. This dish operates on the pleasure principle.

INGREDIENTS

2 cups chopped cherry tomatoes

2 cups chopped broccoli

2 cups chopped, peeled, cucumber

3 tablespoons chopped fresh cilantro

Your favorite no-fat Italian dressing

Salt and pepper to taste

PREPARATION

Mix all vegetables together with cilantro.

Top with a light dose of salad dressing and salt and pepper.

Toss. Done.

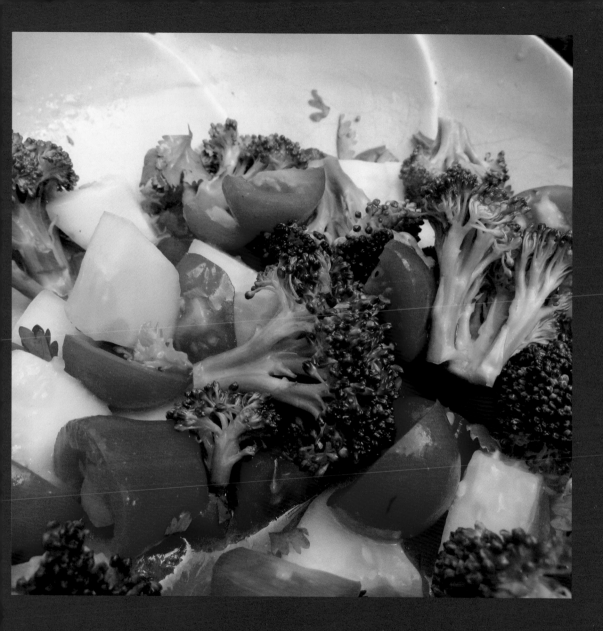

Dates *Phoenix dactylifera*

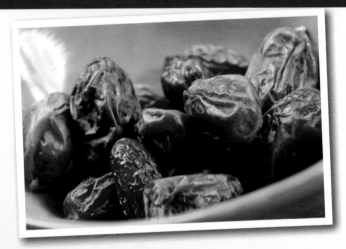

Dark, wrinkly, thick, sultry

*T*HERE ARE MANY FLIRTATIOUS FRUITS IN THE GROCERY STORE THAT ARE seductive, albeit strange. Some are stranger than others – like dates. They are tempting, with their dark, wrinkly, thick, sultry skin, but do you know what to do with one? Go ahead, bite; it's a feast in the form of a sugary chew.

Some accounts record the date palm's cultivation as far back as 6,000 years. In the Bible and the Koran, dates are mentioned with reverence. The Jews considered them a symbol of grace and elegance, often presented as gifts to women. Arabian folklore lists 360 health benefits from this "sacred fruit." In the traditional Hindu diet, dates are a *sattvic* food, giving maximum energy to body and mind.

A date is a real energy powerhouse, loaded with vitamins and minerals – including potassium, which helps with low sperm count in men. And (wouldn't you know) people have long been mixing dates into concoctions as aphrodisiacs, as well as fermenting the date juices into wine.

DATES

Family: Arecaceae

Type: Evergreen palm tree

Color: Yellow orange fruit, foliage green, silver to cream

Harvest Period: Fall

Size: 50 to 100 feet high by 20 to 40 feet wide

Soil: Sand to clay loam

Exposure: Dappled to full sun

Watering: Medium to moist

pH: 4.5 to 8

Cold Hardiness Zone: 9 to 11

Origin: Palm dates have been cultivated for so long – thousands of years – its native origin can only be speculated on. Probably native to the Persian Gulf, northern Africa, the Arabian Peninsula, and northwest India.

Live long and be fertile. The ancient Egyptians used date palm leaves as an emblem of longevity. Hathor, the Egyptian goddess of life, joy, music, dancing, and fertility (note how they all go together) surrounded her sanctuary with a palm grove for easy access.

Why It Works: A Closer Look

But do dates have any real effect on our sex lives and fertility, other than their suggestive appearance? The news is promising. This sweet fruit is believed to have mild estrogen-like effects, increasing the chances of fertility in women. For men, dates may increase sperm count, as well as improve motility. The date contains estradiol and flavonoids, which have a positive effect on sperm quality. Just so you know, some serious studies with male rats showed improved sperm quality and enhanced fertility.

GROWING TIPS

Palm dates, Phoenix dactylifera, are in the Arecaceae family. They no longer grow in the wild and must be cultivated. They are grown mostly on plantations and as ornamental trees in frost-free areas with well-drained soil. Only the female plants produce dates, and only if there is a male nearby. Natural pollination is achieved with the aid of insects or the wind, with the fruits taking six to eight months to ripen. The most common dates available for purchase are 'Medjool' and 'Deglet Noor' (Arabic for "a piece of light").

If you plant a young date palm today, it will bear fruit in three to five years.

Fennel ❧ *Foeniculum vulgare*

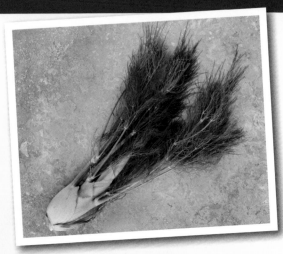

Straight from the Kama Sutra

*F*ENNEL'S REPUTATION THROUGHOUT ANCIENT CULTURES IS PERHAPS PROOF enough of its potency. The *Kama Sutra* of ancient India speaks of fennel as a sexual stimulant. The Egyptians also regarded fennel as an effective libido booster, as did the Chinese. And that's only the beginning of its uses!

A plant that does it all. Every part of the fennel plant – leaves, seeds, and roots – is edible and has long been used for its medicinal value. Our old friend Pliny the Elder (Gaius Plinius Secundus, A.D. 23-79) had so much faith in fennel's medicinal properties that he cited almost two dozen remedies associated with the plant. Due to their sweet scent, fennel seeds were often eaten as breath fresheners, and even today fennel oil is used in perfumes and soaps.

As for fennel's more amorous effects, fennel soup is still served in modern Mediterranean culture to strengthen sexual desire. (Though you certainly don't have to travel that far to prepare it yourself!)

FENNEL

Family: Apiaceae or Umbelliferae

Type: Herbaceous perennial

Color: Green, yellow blooms.

Harvest Period: Summer, June to July

Size: 3 to 5 feet high and 2 to 3 feet wide

Soil: Moist, well-drained

Exposure: Full sun

Watering: Medium

pH: 6 to 7

Cold Hardiness Zone: 4 to 9

Origin: Indigenous to Mediterranean shores, but has become widely naturalized in many parts of the world, especially near the seacoast and on riverbanks.

Why It Works: A Closer Look

Fennel stimulates the effects of estrogen to increase libido in women. Don't feel too left out though, guys – fennel has also been known to increase testosterone, relieving male menopause and impotence.

Frankly, there should be a warning label on this plant. Fennel comes at you from so many directions there is no escaping its magical spell. Its pheromones, phytoestro-gens, and an estrogen-like substance called estragole can boost your sensual side. Not to mention its wide host of vitamins and nutrients to keep your sex life healthy! Even fennel oil's sweet aroma can act as an arousal aid for women.

Little testing has confirmed fennel's aphrodisiac attributes on humans, but a study in the 1980s showed an elevated libido in male and female rats. In the 1930s, fennel was found to be so rich in phytoestrogens that it was considered a synthetic source of estrogen. So maybe our ancestors were onto something after all… ✀

GROWING TIPS

Fennel, Foeniculum vulgare, is a member of the Apiaceae (or Umbelliferae) family, which includes other aromatic plants such as caraway, cilantro, cumin and Queen Anne's lace.

Fennel is so easily grown that it is considered invasive throughout the United States. It grows best in full sun and moist, organically-rich, well-drained soils. Because fennel re-seeds freely, remove the flowers before they go to seed to stop the plant from overtaking your garden.

Fun fact: fennel also attracts swallowtail butterflies, so you may make some new friends in your garden as well!

Fennel and Onion Marmalade

From the kitchen of
Carolyn Binder,
Cowlick Cottage Farm

Makes 2-plus cups

Earthy and grown underground in the shadow of the soil, root vegetables possess a certain mystique. Here's a sweet and savory side that will have you dishing your date seconds.

INGREDIENTS

1 tablespoon olive oil

1 medium sweet onion, thinly sliced

1 large fennel, thinly sliced, fronds reserved for garnish

1 cup demerara sugar

1 cup white balsamic vinegar

Salt and pepper, to taste

PREPARATION

In a cast iron skillet, warm olive oil over medium heat.

Add the onion and cook for 2 minutes.

Add the fennel and cook another 2 minutes.

Add sugar and vinegar. Cook for 20 minutes or until marmalade thickens.

Season with salt and pepper, and garnish with fennel fronds.

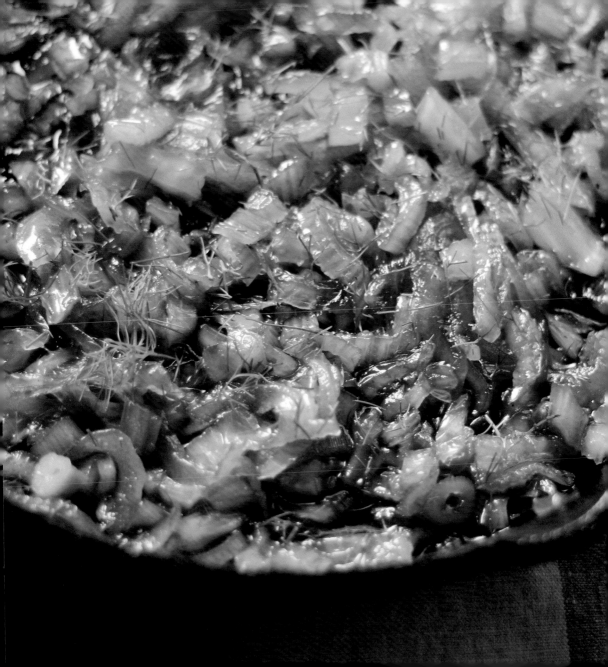

Fig ❧ *Ficus carica*

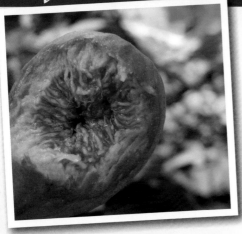

The apple...
or the fig?

*O*N MID TO LATE SUMMER, MY FIG TREE IS AS POPULAR AS A BORROWED BEACH house! For a few weeks each year, my figs ripen for a rustic luxury no other fruit can equal – plucked fresh from the tree. Enjoying each sweet bite, I'm reminded why I grow this beast of a fruit. The common fig tree, and its many cultivars selected from the species, can grow to incredible sizes. Despite its bulk, however, the fig tree is a worthwhile investment. While dried varieties can be purchased year round, fresh figs are hard to come by.

A very...aesthetic appeal. The aphrodisiac power of figs stems from its sexual appearance, flavor, texture and fragrance, which together can heighten our senses. Through the ages, figs have been associated with increasing sexual stamina, improving mood, and waking up the libido.

Adam and Eve in the Bible wore fig leaves to cover themselves after their fall from grace. There are some scholars who even believe it was the fig that tempted Eve, not the apple. The Greeks were introduced to the enticing fruit in the 9th century B.C., but the Romans believed

FIG

Family: Moraceae

Type: Showy, edible fruit

Color: Green leaves with fruit color dependent on type

Harvest Period: A short season, midsummer

Size: 10 to 20 feet high and wide

Soil: Wide range

Exposure: Full sun to part shade

Watering: Medium

pH: 5.5 to 8, but 6 to 6.5 is ideal

Cold Hardiness Zone: 8 to 9, and protected areas including 6 and 7

Origin: Western Asia and Eastern Mediterranean

it was Bacchus, god of wine, revelry and fertility, who introduced the fig to mankind. So it's really no surprise that the fig earned a reputation as an aphrodisiac.

The fig was also said to be Cleopatra's favorite food. I can't blame her, since its voluptuous shape, succulent chew, and honey-scented taste does take you away for a moment. Or two. Bite into one and you'll see.

Why It Works: A Closer Look

Packed with potassium, manganese, anti-oxidants, amino acids, and the highest mineral content of all common fruits, figs also support proper pH levels in the body. This makes it more difficult for pathogens to invade, so you're always feeling your best – and a healthier body makes for a healthier love life!

Nutritional value aside, there doesn't appear to be much science to support claims about the fig's aphrodisiac properties. Nonetheless, it's been considered a visual sexual stimulus for centuries – and it's certainly hard to argue with perception. If your mind goes there, it's an aphrodisiac. ✄

GROWING TIPS

Figs are typically grown in subtropical regions, but can also thrive in areas with warmer winters, or if kept in a sheltered location.

Interestingly, fig trees don't show visible blossoms before fruiting. What we think of as fruit are actually drupelets, or flowers that have inverted inward. Because figs do not keep well, they should be harvested ripe from the tree when you intend to use them.

Fig-licious Appetizer

Yield: 8 slices/wedges

As an organic gardener practicing sustainable methods, I never worry about eating a fig fresh from the tree. Simple, seductive and sensual, the fig needs no embellishment. But for those times when you want to charm the pants off someone, elevate the status of the fig with this easy to make appetizer.

INGREDIENTS

2 slices cooked, chopped bacon

4 ounces crumbled goat cheese, softened

1 tablespoon finely chopped toasted pecans (*toasting instructions below)

1 teaspoon chopped fresh thyme

12 fresh figs, sliced lengthwise

1 tablespoon honey

6 toasted baguette slices, if desired

PREPARATION

Preheat oven to 350° F.
Stir together chopped bacon, goat cheese, toasted pecans and thyme.

Cut figs in half. Press the back of a small spoon into the center of each of the fig halves, making a small indentation in each.

Spoon the bacon and cheese mixture into the indentations.

Bake on a greased baking sheet for 7 minutes.

Drizzle the still-warm figs with honey.
Serve immediately with toasted baguette slices, if desired, or just on their own.

*To toast pecans: Preheat oven to 350°F. Spread pecans on a baking sheet and place in the oven to toast, just until they become aromatic, about 5 minutes. Stir every minute or so.

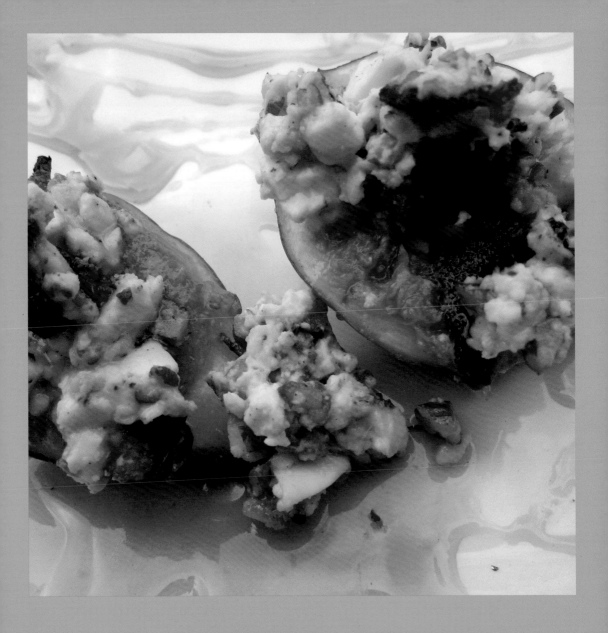

Garlic ❦ *Allium sativum*

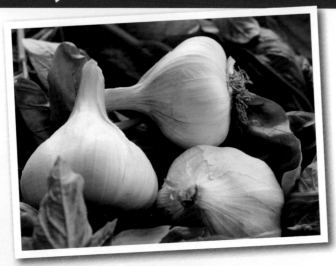

Keep your distance… no, I mean come closer!

ARLIC!? YES GARLIC, THAT BULB WITH SUCH AN ALLURING SCENT, ALSO becomes a vile stink if both of you aren't eating it. Since Greek and Roman times, garlic has been known as the stinking rose. It's the last food you should think of eating prior to meeting your date if you're hoping for a successful evening; if you both partake, then no harm done – in fact, just the opposite.

I'll admit, it does seem odd that a stinky bulb can stimulate passions to the extent that it does. Garlic has a long reputation for increasing sexual drive. In India, the ancient Laws of Manu forbade the eating of garlic by Brahmins because it stirred the passions. Today, many Eastern celibate orders, including Tibetan Buddhist monks, abstain from garlic for the same reason.

GARLIC

Family: Alliaceae

Type: Bulb

Color: Green tops, white bulbs

Harvest Period: Summer

Size: 1 to 1.5 feet high by 0.75 to 1 feet wide

Soil: Well-drained soil

Exposure: Full sun

Watering: Medium

pH: 6 to 7

Cold Hardiness Zone: 4 to 9

Origin: Not known in the wild

Oh, if you insist. On the other hand, we have the Prophet Ezra to thank for commanding the eating of garlic on the eve of the Sabbath, to ensure the mitzvah of conjugal pleasure. Garlic is mentioned elsewhere in the Bible, the Talmud and in Homer's *Odyssey*. Certainly an important herb for those times, as well as useful today.

Garlic lore tells us that the bulb protects against vampires. If I were an individual study, I could prove the claim, because despite all the vampire movies I've watched and books I've read to keep up with my teenage daughters, I've never had to deal with a vampire directly. Clearly it works.

Why It Works: A Closer Look

Garlic is well known for its powerful antibiotic properties, something Louis Pasteur and others since have attested to. In Russia it's called "the Russian penicillin." Garlic is considered a "hot" herb. But garlic's aphrodisiac bona fides come from the fact that it improves blood circulation. Anything that gets the blood going can improve sexual performance in men. It's a recurring theme in aphrodisiac awareness. ✀

GROWING TIPS

Growing garlic is easy enough. I grow mine in a container. This works well for people who have a sunny balcony and must grow plants in pots.

In fall or spring, plant bulbets 2 inches deep in organically rich, well-drained soil with medium moisture. The pointed end should be facing up. Harvest in early or late summer (depending on your location) after the leaves turn brown and begin to fall over. Dry bulbs for several days before storing in a cool, dry location.

Roasted Garlic Butter

From the kitchen of
Carolyn Binder,
Cowlick Cottage Farm

Yield: 1¼ cup

Roasted garlic makes a better butter. No doubt if butter were a plant, it would top the list of aphrodisiacs. Julia Child knew this well. Anything that can give that much pleasure is an aphrodisiac of the first order! So if we can't bring the butter to the aphrodisiac plant list, let's bring the aphrodisiac to the butter. Eat roasted garlic butter responsibly.

INGREDIENTS

1 cup butter, softened

1 tablespoon or more minced,
roasted garlic*

¼ cup grated aged Parmesan cheese

1 tablespoon kosher salt

1 teaspoon Italian seasoning
or garden herbs

½ teaspoon freshly ground black pepper

¼ teaspoon cayenne pepper
(optional, but good!)

PREPARATION

Mix all recipe ingredients together in the food processor bowl and pulse a couple of times to blend.

Slather it on bread and broil. Melt it on grilled steaks. Drizzle it on steamed vegetables. Use it as a dip for fresh lobster or crab. Be humble when accepting compliments.

*To roast garlic: Cut off the top ½ inch of a head of garlic and drizzle with olive oil. Wrap tightly in foil and roast in a 400°F oven for half an hour or until the cloves are soft and popping out of the top of the garlic skins. Freshly harvested garlic may take 5-10 minutes longer to roast. Let cool to room temperature. Refrigerate or continue with the recipe.

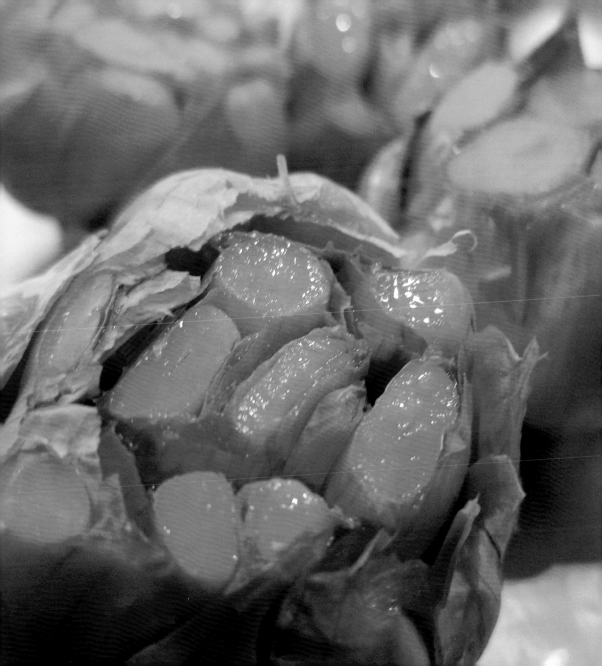

Ginger Root ❦ *Zingiber officinale*

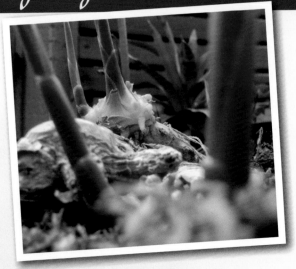

Warning: will provoke lust

GINGER IS THE WORLD'S MOST WIDELY CULTIVATED HERB. AS EARLY AS 500 B.C., Confucius wrote about its excellent digestive merits, remarking that he was never without ginger. Alexander the Great brought ginger back from India to Greece where, later, Dioscorides recommended it for cooking and to calm and benefit the stomach.

That's all well and good, you say, but what about, you know, the "benefits"?

Ginger's aphrodisiac qualities have been written about in Chinese and Indian cultures for thousands of years. Once the plant came west, there was no stopping it. Avicenna, the 11th century Persian physician wrote that ginger "heightens lustful thoughts." In Italy, the famed medieval medical school of Salerno prescribed a cure for aging men who had lost their vigor: "Eat ginger and you will love and be loved as in your youth." In the 16th century, English apothecarist John Gerard was worried about the benefits of ginger, saying it was provoking lust. I can only imagine the rise in sales after that warning.

GINGER ROOT

Family: Zingiberaceae

Type: Herbaceous perennial, culinary herb, suitable for annual

Color: Leathery root

Harvest Period: About four months into the growing season. Roots are near the surface, and can be cut as needed. At the end of the season, when the leaves fade, the entire root can be lifted and stored for later use.

Size: 2 to 4 feet high and wide

Soil: Fertile, well-drained

Exposure: Part shade

Watering: Medium to wet

pH: 6.1 to 6.5

Cold Hardiness Zone: 9 to 12

Origin: Tropical Asia

Putting the moves on. It is said that sperm are helped along with ginger, a natural fertility booster, increasing motility and viability. Ginger may help invigorate the reproductive organs and even assist with impotence and premature ejaculation. I'm blushing now. "Honey, fancy some sushi tonight?" Skip the fish and ask for extra helpings of ginger to cleanse your palate.

Why It Works: A Closer Look

Referred to as "The Universal Medicine" in Ayurveda (India's 5,000-year-old Science of Life), ginger works to stimulate the heart and circulation, enhancing blood flow.

Ginger has a characteristic taste and smell; used in a tea, it has a warming effect that is felt throughout the body, including the reproductive system, for men and women. Next time you need a lift, sip a hot cup of ginger tea a few times during the day and see if it doesn't just lift your mood.

GROWING TIPS

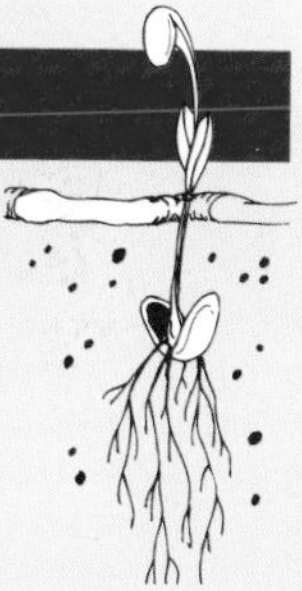

A tropical plant, ginger is easy to grow if you have enough heat and humidity. My Raleigh garden has the humidity but not enough heat year-round, so I grow it as an annual, or most often, I buy what I need from the Asian market.

Plant the fresh ginger root. Ginger is convenient when grown in pots – a great balcony plant if you have part shade. Plant fresh ginger purchased from the grocery store in early spring. Dried or frozen won't work; it needs to be fresh.

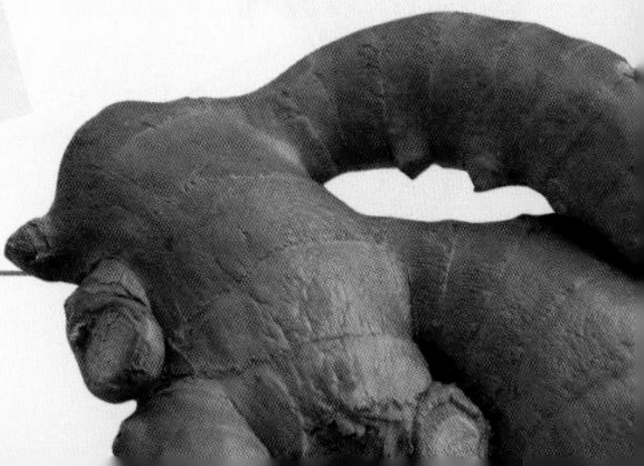

Ginger Shortbread

From the kitchen of Steve Asbell

Yield: 8 slices/wedges

Some of my favorite flavors are shortbread and ginger, but before I tried Steve's recipe, I'd never had them together, and certainly not with cardamom! This recipe will give you a new perspective on adding aphrodisiacs to an otherwise mild-mannered cookie. Break the mold and let the fun begin!

INGREDIENTS

¼ cup crystallized (candied) ginger, finely chopped

1 ½ cups all-purpose flour

3 tablespoons granulated sugar

1 tablespoon ground cardamom

½ cup cold butter

1 tablespoon cinnamon

PREPARATION

Preheat oven to 325°F.
Combine chopped ginger with flour, sugar and cardamom in a bowl. (If you don't have crystallized ginger, substitute one tablespoon fresh grated ginger mixed with one tablespoon sugar.) Stir ginger, flour, sugar and cardamom together.

Add a stick of cold butter and, using a blender, mix in until the dough is fine and crumbly. Then knead the mixture together until it makes a smooth ball.

Place the ball of dough on an ungreased cookie sheet and shape it into a seven-inch circle. Cut the dough into eight even wedges.

Bake for 25 minutes or until the edges start to brown. Slice the wedges again, garnish with cinnamon and allow the shortbread to cool before serving.

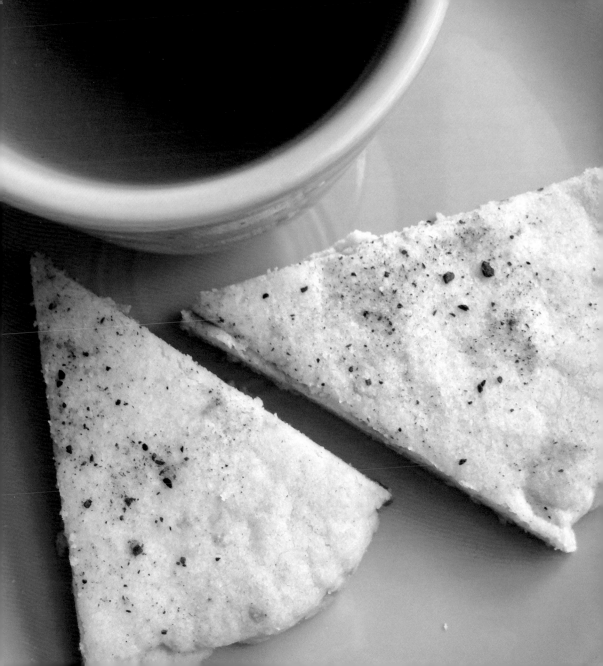

Ginseng 🌿 *Panax quinquefolius*

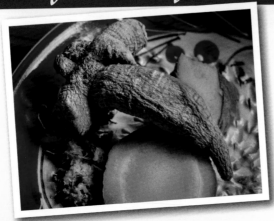

It's a yin and yang thing

𝒯HE HERBAL SUPPLEMENT FOLKS ARE QUICK TO SELL YOU A PILL FOR WHAT AILS you. Many of us dutifully follow along. But the root of the ginseng plant has an impressive 5,000-year-old track record to attest to its energizing claims.

There are a few kinds of ginseng, so don't confuse the American ginseng, *Panax quinquefolius* with the Asian ginseng, *Panax ginseng;* both, however, are considered powerful rejuvenators. Panax is derived from the Greek *panakeia* (panacea), which translates to "universal remedy;" the word ginseng comes from the Chinese term *jen-shen*, meaning "man-root."

Asians have long revered the ginseng plant for its restorative powers to enhance vitality and sex drive in both men and women, believing that if taken for a long time, it strengthens the body and extends life. The Koreans have even fed ginseng root to their racehorses for better performance.

Ginseng yin and yang. Over time, it was discovered that the power of Asian ginseng became better when blended with American ginseng. According to Traditional Chinese Medicine, things living in cold places (Asia) are strong in yang, and things living in hot places

GINSENG

Family: Araliaceae

Type: Herbaceous perennial

Color: Whitish root

Harvest Period: At maturity (7 to 10 years)

Size: 0.75 to 1.5 feet high and wide

Soil: Rich, high-humus, well-drained soil.

Exposure: Part shade to full shade

Watering: Medium

pH: 5 to 6

Cold Hardiness Zone: 4 to 8

Origin: Eastern North America

(much of North America) are strong in yin. As such, the two together are balanced. Yang energy is hot, positive and male, while yin energy is cool, negative and female – the positive and negative, referring to polarity rather than character.

Asian panax is found to improve circulation and increase blood supply.

American ginseng cleanses excess yang from the body, bringing calmness. The two together are in balance.

Why It Works: A Closer Look

In part, the aphrodisiac benefit of ginseng has to do with appearances. Ginseng root looks very much like the human body part (remember, it's the "man-root").

But recently, a 2002 animal study by the Southern Illinois University School of Medicine, researching both forms of ginseng, added new evidence to the growing support for the use of ginseng in the treatment of sexual dysfunction. ✄

GROWING TIPS

American ginseng is in the Araliaceae family, also known as the Aralia family, which includes ivy, celery, and carrots. Asian ginseng is considered close cousins with the American variety probably finding its way to North American over the ancient land bridge between Siberia and Alaska.

Grow ginseng by directly sowing seeds in the fall, after the leaves have fallen. Select a moist, well-shaded site, under a deciduous tree. Be patient though, it can take 7 to 10 years for your plants to mature. You can harvest ginseng then, but if left to grow, this long-lived plant can be left for your children's children's children.

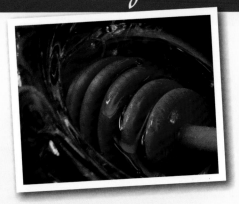

Why Cupid dipped his arrows in honey

A TRUE GIFT FROM NATURE HERSELF, HONEY HAS EARNED ITS TITLE AS THE nectar of the gods.

Since before recorded time, bees have been prominent in the lives of mankind, as evident in an 8,000 year-old Spanish cave painting depicting a man riding a wild honeybee nest, and others showing honey-gathers climbing trees to harvest honey from wild bees. Similar ancient drawings have been found in Africa, Asia, India and Australia. Later, honey was one of the first foods named in the 4th millennium Sumerian and Babylonian cuneiform writings, the Hittite code, and the sacred writings of India and Egypt. In fact, you'd be hard-pressed to find a culture that didn't treasure honey for its healing and vitality benefits.

The Egyptians used honey to cure sterility and impotence. The ancient Greeks associated bees and honey with fertility and childbirth, and one of the depictions of the goddess Artemis shows her as half woman, half bee. Cupid, that trickster, dipped his arrows in honey before aiming at lovers. During medieval times, mead, a popular honeyed drink was drunk to "sweeten" a honeymoon. Honey is mentioned as an aphrodisiac in both the *Kama Sutra* and the 15th-century Arabic sex manual and work of erotic literature, *The Perfumed Garden of Sensual Delights*. It wasn't a secret.

WHITE CLOVER

Featured Plant: White clover, *Trifolium repens*

Family: Fabaceae

Type: Perennial

Color: White flowers

Harvest Period: Spring

Size: 3 inches high and 12 inches wide

Soil: Well-drained, fertile soils

Exposure: Full sun

Watering: Medium

pH: 6 to 7

Cold Hardiness Zone: Through zone 4

Origin: Europe, North Africa, and West Asia

Who knew? Augustus, Aristotle, Benjamin Franklin, George Washington, Thomas Jefferson and Leo Tolstoy were all beekeepers. Even Martha Stewart and the White House host hives.

Why It Works: A Closer Look

A healer of the body in many ways, honey also contributes to our sexual wellbeing. It is rich in B vitamins, enzymes, and amino acids and is widely believed to promote virility and reproductive health. It stimulates the growth and regeneration of body tissues and the formation of red blood cells.

Eating honey regularly increases the production, quality and motility of sperm cells. The chemical chrysin promotes testosterone production in men, and the mineral boron aids estrogen production in women. One study found that a three-ounce dose of honey "significantly increased the level of nitric oxide," the chemical released in the blood during arousal in both men and women. ✀

GROWING TIPS

White clover, Trifolium repens, is thought of as a living mulch, planted between crop rows, fruit bushes and trees. The flower attracts bees and other beneficial insects to pollinate plants.

White clover produces above-ground stolons (creeping stems) that root at the nodes and quickly fill in large areas. Clover is a great addition to the urban lawn, and at one time was a staple in grass seed mixtures. If you become a beekeeper (and I hope to this year) growing clover in your lawn will make your bees very happy indeed.

Feel Good Tea

From the kitchen of
Carolyn Binder,
Cowlick Cottage Farm

**Makes 8 ounces
of flavored honey
to use in 16 cups of tea**

I made Carolyn's honey-based Feel Good Tea and fell in love with the first sip. It's a staple in my fridge now for a quick pick-me-up. This combination of honey, ginger and lemon might just become your go-to restorative.

INGREDIENTS

1 cup local, organic honey

1 organic lemon, washed and sliced, ends discarded

Several slices of peeled, fresh organic ginger

PREPARATION

Fill a pretty jar about halfway with the honey. Add lemon and ginger slices, alternating them. Top off with additional honey, leaving a half-inch of headspace. Store in the refrigerator, letting it steep for a few days before using it. Stir gently before serving.

Add one tablespoon of flavored honey to a teacup and top with boiling water. Ahhh…

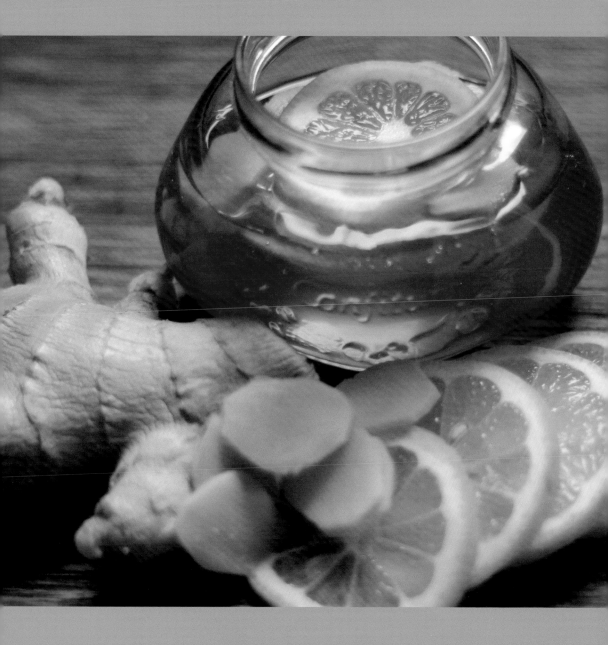

Beekeeping

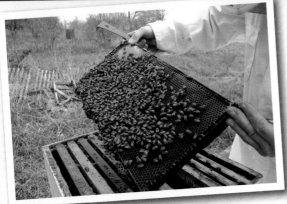

EES HAVE BEEN KEPT FOR 4,000 YEARS. Before that, people braved wild nests in trees or on the sides of cliffs. The prize? Honey. Sweet, golden honey...nectar of the gods.

How do they do it? Bees do not actually create honey; they improve upon a plant product – nectar. It takes two million bee trips to flowers to produce one pound of honey. A single bee visits between 50 and 100 flowers a day, collecting about half its body weight in pollen, In its six-week lifetime, a bee will only contribute up to ^{1}/12th-teaspoon of honey. The business of being a bee is not easy.

Urban beekeeping is on the rise in response to the reports of colony-collapse disorder, a recent crisis in which large populations of honeybees suddenly die. To do our part for the bees (and other wildlife), pesticide-free, sustainable gardening practices are a must. I plan to have bees because I can. I welcome them – and birds and other wildlife – into my pesticide-free garden. I want to provide a safe area for their survival. It's important to support all bees in our gardens, the honey-making bees along with the native bees. Both are equally important.

The wild nature of the honeybee, or *Apis mellifera*, is part of the fascination of beekeeping. However, we are able to "tame" them to some extent, using modern beekeeping systems with movable frames that make harvesting honey easy. These hives are used by beekeeping enthusiasts in urban gardens, suburbs, and even on rooftops of high-rise buildings. In other parts of the world, ancient methods like the traditional mud hives in Egypt are still in use today.

There are countless clubs and online groups to guide you in the ancient craft of beekeeping. It's an exciting and satisfying way to become a better steward of the land. And just think of all that honey!

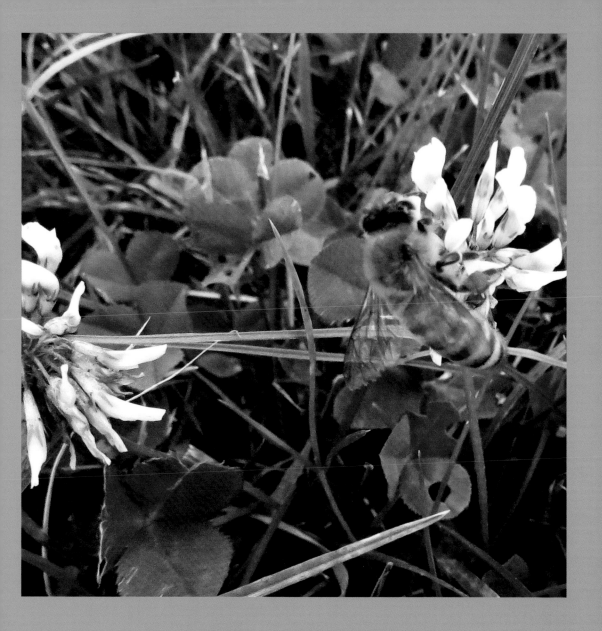

Common Jasmine ❧ *Jasminum officinale*

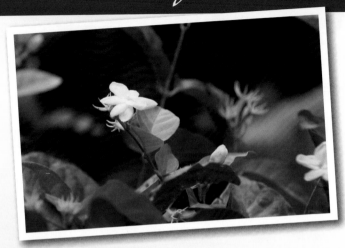

The perfume of love

𝒯HE SCENT OF THE JASMINE ON A SUMMER EVENING BREEZE IS SO DELIGHTFUL that it's impossible to not feel romantic as you pass by this tangled vine.

Even the name has an exotic feel. Native to Mediterranean countries, Asia Minor, the Himalayas and China, its name *jasmine* is derived from the Persian word *yasmin*, meaning "god's gift." Jasmine has been used as an aphrodisiac for centuries in China, the Arabian Peninsula, and India. In traditional Hindu culture jasmine is known as the "perfume of love," and even today, the nuptial beds of newlyweds are decorated with the flowers of this sweet-smelling plant.

But it's not all about the scent. While the aroma of jasmine drifting on the evening air is unmistakably intoxicating, there are other benefits to this plant as well. Sipping jasmine tea has been known to revitalize and restore energy, soothe nerves, and produce a feeling of confidence. Jasmine tea is easily prepared by adding flowers to oolong or green tea. Steep, then strain the flowers. And don't forget to relax…

JASMINE

Family: Oleaceae

Type: Vine

Color: White, pink

Harvest Period: Seasonal bloomer, spring through fall

Size: 20 to 30 feet high and 7 to 15 feet wide

Soil: Fertile, well-drained

Exposure: Full sun to part shade

Watering: Medium

pH: A wide range, between 4.9 and 8.4

Cold Hardiness Zone: 8 to 10

Origin: Asia Minor, Himalayas, China, India

Because of its restorative properties, jasmine has traditionally been used for sexual problems such as impotence and premature ejaculation in men and lack of desire in women. Try using jasmine oil for a massage or diluted in the bath to ease tension, stress and nerves.

Why It Works: A Closer Look

Although jasmine's sweet, sultry scent acts strongly on our romantic imaginations, there is not much science to support its aphrodisiac reputation. Chemical components such as jasmone and benzyl acetate create the smell and flavor in jasmine and its essential oils that relax the body, making a cup of jasmine tea or a bit of aromatherapy the perfect way to calm your nerves before – or after – a date night.

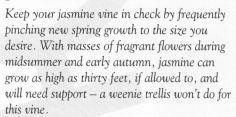

GROWING TIPS

Common jasmine, Jasminum officinale, is a member of the Oleaceae family. It grows best in warmer climates (zone 8 and above), but can also winter inside if removed before the first frost, or be grown as an annual.

Keep your jasmine vine in check by frequently pinching new spring growth to the size you desire. With masses of fragrant flowers during midsummer and early autumn, jasmine can grow as high as thirty feet, if allowed to, and will need support – a weenie trellis won't do for this vine.

Jasmine flowers have the strongest scent in the evening. Plant it where you can enjoy the fragrance most, such as the back porch where you sit and relax after dinner, or perhaps around your bedroom window, where the scent can drift in on the soothing summer air.

Lavender ✿ *Lavandula augustifolia*

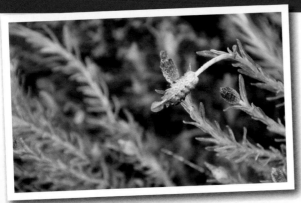

Five stars from the Queen of Sheba

*L*AVENDER, LOVE, AND SEDUCTION HAVE LONG BEEN INTERTWINED IN OUR cultural imagination. From biblical times onward, lavender shows up in the lives of famous people, often for the purpose of getting someone into bed. The Queen of Sheba anointed herself with lavender and other fragrant oils to capture King Solomon's heart. Judith anointed herself with lavender to seduce Holofernes and thus save Jerusalem from destruction. And Cleopatra famously doused herself with lavender (her favorite love potion) to bring Julius Caesar and Marc Antony to heel.

In Tudor times, it was tradition to place lavender under the beds of newlyweds to invite passion. We're told that Josephine gave Napoleon Bonaparte a drink that was filled with lavender flowers to keep his fidelity. Perhaps Napoleon should have given the drink to Josephine, for she was not loyal to him.

Lavender lures. Long before lavender sachets, women would scent their clothes, linens, and trousseau with sprigs of lavender. Lavender, added to teas and bath water, was always the scent of choice to promote fidelity within a love union; few things are more alluring than loyalty from our partner.

LAVENDER

Family: Lamiacea

Type: Herbaceous perennial

Color: Fragrant, purple blooms

Harvest Period: Spring

Size: 1 to 1.5 feet high and wide

Soil: Gritty, or sandy loam

Exposure: Full sun

Watering: Dry to medium

pH: 6 to 8

Cold Hardiness Zone: 5 to 8

Origin: Mediterranean

Today, lavender oils are used to help promote restful sleep, relieve tension headaches and ease muscle pains, and it is still used as an aphrodisiac. Our foremothers were right: lavender lures men.

Why It Works: A Closer Look

A study conducted by the Smell & Taste Treatment Research Foundation in Chicago exposed men to a variety of food aromas and then graded the level of their sexual arousal by measuring the blood flow to their genital regions. Lavender (in combination with pumpkin) measured a 40% increase in blood flow. This is significant when compared to cheese pizza, which only showed an increase of 5%, or buttered popcorn at 9%.

Clearly, we should be adding lavender to our pizza, and seasoning popcorn with this herb. ✀

GROWING TIPS

Common lavender, Lavandula angustifolia – or English lavender – is a versatile perennial in the Lamiacea family, along with other aromatics such as basil, mint, rosemary, and sage. It grows best in a sunny location with average to dry, well-drained, alkaline soil and full sun.

It will help to know the right lavender for your garden. For my garden in Raleigh, N.C., an area of high humidity and rainfall, I've found better success growing Spanish lavender, Lavandula stoechas. Their cultures are similar, but I find the flowers on the English lavender to be much prettier.

Interestingly, English lavender isn't native to England, but comes primarily from the Mediterranean region, yet it has adapted well to the English countryside. Considered "true lavender", English lavender is what is used in essential oils from which sprays and aromatherapy oils are made.

Lavender Cookies

From the kitchen of Lily Philbrook

Yield: 2 dozen cookies

As we learned from the chapter on lavender, this plant has benefits! If you do nothing else, spray your bed linens with a lavender-infused mist. (Close your eyes, Lily.) And I personally approve the eating of these lavender cookies in bed.

(P.S. Lily is my 13-year-old daughter. See her thoughts on cooking with flowers, below left.)

INGREDIENTS

1¼ sticks of butter

½ cup white sugar

1 egg

1 tablespoon lavender flowers, plus 1 tablespoon to top after cooking

1½ cups all-purpose flour

Lily Says: Cooking is one of my two passions. My other passion is writing. When I cook with ingredients that come from my own home, it adds more meaning to the product. Lavender is a flower that can be used everywhere in cooking: on eggs, on fish, and on cookies! These cookies do not taste very sugary, for it is the lavender that gives them flavor. As you bite into a cookie, close your eyes and imagine a new world. Taste the lavender in every bite, and I hope it brings you to your garden. Enjoy!

PREPARATION

Preheat oven to 350 °F. Grease cookie sheets.

Cream the butter and sugar together. Beat the egg, and blend it into the butter and sugar. Mix in the lavender flowers and the flour. Drop batter by teaspoonfuls onto cookie sheets.

Bake 15 to 20 minutes, or until golden. Remove cookies to cooling racks; sprinkle additional lavender flowers, if desired.

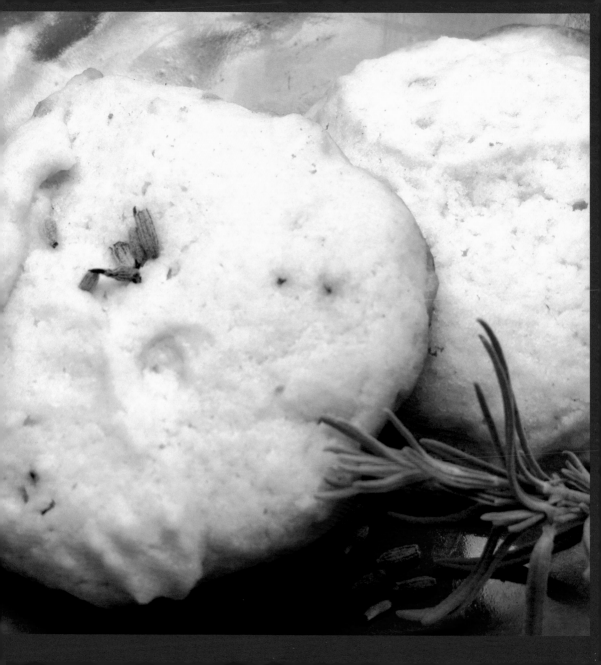

Licorice Root ❧ *Glycyrrhiza glabra*

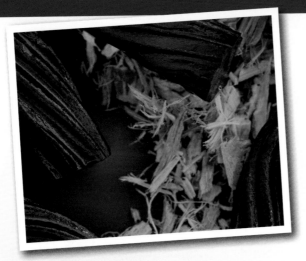

Mixed messages for the male libido

*I*S LICORICE ROOT AN APHRODISIAC? A QUALIFIED YES, BUT THE SCIENCE ABOUT this herb is a bit conflicted on the topic.

A little popularity goes a long way. Licorice root has been used for medical and symbolic purposes for centuries. The Egyptians must have prized it highly, because not only was it found in the tomb of King Tut, but ancient hieroglyphs reveal that men commonly consumed a beverage made from the root. In the Hindu tradition, the *Kama Sutra* includes several licorice-based recipes for increasing sexual vigor. Our Roman friends considered licorice root an important aid in maintaining male vitality and physical stamina. It was also commonly used in traditional Chinese medicine, and even today is the second most-prescribed herb in China, behind ginseng. Licorice made its way to Europe during the Middle Ages and was eventually introduced to the Native Americans for its medicinal properties. In pagan cultures, crushed licorice root was used in love sachets and in spells to ensure fidelity. Sweet, right? Well, there

LICORICE ROOT

Family: Fabaceae

Type: Herbaceous perennial

Color: Grayish green

Harvest Period: Autumn

Size: 4 feet high and 3 wide

Soil: Well-drained

Exposure: Full sun

Watering: Moist

pH: 4 to 8

Cold Hardiness Zone: 8a

Origin: Southern Europe, Middle East, and parts of Asia

actually may have been an ulterior motive to these little gifts (and this is where it gets complicated). Read on.

Why It Works: A Closer Look

Despite the common association of licorice root with sexuality, a study published in the New England Journal of Medicine concluded that licorice root actually *suppresses* libido by interfering with testosterone production.

So why am I writing about licorice root if it has the opposite effect of enticing love?

Because another study, by neurologist Alan Hirsch, M.D., concluded that the smell of a certain popular licorice candy dramatically stimulated the male libido, increasing the blood flow to the penis by thirteen percent. And get this: the combined scent of black licorice and doughnuts increased flow by thirty-two percent. Hmm. So maybe it's really the smell that gets us excited. No wonder the "Hot Doughnuts Now" sign at our local Krispy Kreme is such a popular draw! ✄

GROWING TIPS

Licorice root, Glycyrrhiza glabra, *is a member of the legume family of plants and is easy to grow. Licorice root grows best in a sunny location on sandy soil in moist locations. The roots are double, with a taproot and horizontal rhizomes. Harvest the licorice root by digging up the plant and cutting away the crown.*

If you are so inclined, licorice root brews nicely into an herbal tea. Add approximately 1 teaspoon of chopped or freshly grated licorice root to a cup of hot water. Steep for 10 to 15 minutes, then strain. But remember, you may actually experience, shall we say, a calming effect. Don't say I didn't warn you.

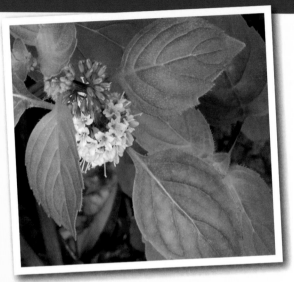

Will inspire kissing

*I*F YOU WERE A GEEKY FAN OF GREEK MYTHOLOGY IN HIGH SCHOOL, LIKE I WAS, you'll never tire of tales about mythical gods and nymphs and spells cast on those that did them wrong. Even if you weren't a fan, you might like to learn about Menthe.

The tale begins with Hades, the god of the Underworld. Hades had a love affair with the river nymph Menthe. When Hades' wife, Persephone, got wind of the relationship between her husband and Menthe, she didn't take too kindly to it. With all her power, she cast a spell upon Menthe and turned her into a plant – what we know today as mint. Now Menthe would forever be crushed beneath the feet of passersby. But Hades to the rescue. Though unable to reverse the spell completely, he was able give his beloved the power to sweeten the air whenever anyone stepped upon her. And so she does, as a testament to their love.

APPLE MINT

Featured plant: Apple Mint

Family: Lamiaceae

Type: Herbaceous perennial, suitable as an annual

Color: Mint green

Harvest Period: Pinch leaves for use anytime they are present

Size: 1 to 2 feet high and wide

Soil: Rich, moist, organic soil.

Exposure: Full sun to part shade

Watering: Medium to wet

pH: 6 to 7.5

Cold Hardiness Zone: 5 to 9

Origin: Southern and western Europe

Nature's freshener. There were several uses of mint throughout history, from the Greeks adding it to their baths to stimulate their bodies to the Romans chewing on fresh leaves as a mouth freshener. The Greeks would also scrub down the banquet tables with mint for a refreshing preparation prior to meals. I tried this at home, and it's amazing the feeling it presented. Everything was, well, fresh. As to the sexiness of mint, it may also have mildly aphrodisiac benefits.

Why It Works: A Closer Look

The enticing aroma of menthol, an essential oil found in mint leaves, works the senses. Considered a psychological enhancer, mint's aroma has a calming effect. There is actually a study that says mint on your breath will inspire kissing. I would suggest trying this at home.

Mint also contains several vitamins and minerals important to maintaining good sexual health, including A and C and trace amounts of B2, calcium, copper, magnesium, potassium and zinc. Personally, I think it's more about that sweet, fresh smell and the nymph Menthe's desire to bring your relaxation to the next level. ✂

GROWING TIPS

Apple mint, Mentha suaveolens, is a member of the Lamiaceae family, keeping company with other aroma aphrodisiacs such as basil, rosemary, thyme and lavender and other mints, of course.

As with most mints, apple mint can be aggressive, its underground stems (rhizomes) sending out roots and shoots from its nodes. Best if grown with barrier borders or in containers. The leaves make an excellent tea or addition to salads and baths.

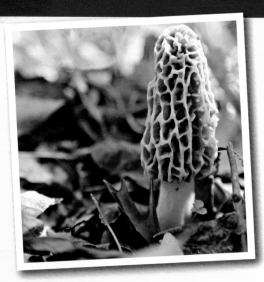

Dangerously sexy

MUSHROOMS IN GENERAL ARE SOMEWHAT OF AN ENIGMA, OFTEN SPROUTING up fully-grown overnight as if by magic. As for taste, they're either loved or loathed – commonly because of fear of possible poisoning. There are many toxic look-alikes in the wild that make it dangerous to just pop a 'shroom in our mouths. We humans often go to great lengths to fire up the libido, though, and there are some mushrooms out there that do just that.

Like them or not, mushrooms get around. The Hebrews believed that God provided the Israelites (Exodus 16:1-36) with "manna from heaven" in the form of fungus. Some ancient cultures thought of mushrooms as gifts the gods left after a lightning strike, which actually isn't too far from the truth. Mushrooms can grow from the ashes of fire, as was evident after the Mt. St. Helens eruption in 1980. An 8th century B.C. Greek vase depicts unusual mushrooms at the feet of one of the famous Centaurs, Nessus; it was believed that the centaurs' antics were enhanced by this potent fungus.

MUSHROOM/MOREL

Featured Plant: Morels, *Morchella esculenta*

Family: Morchellaceae

Type: Fungi

Color: Grayish brown

Harvest Period: Early spring

Size: 0.75 to 3 inches high and 0.75 to 4 inches wide

Soil: Nutrient-rich soil that freezes over in winter

Exposure: Shade

Watering: Moist

pH: 6.4

Cold Hardiness Zone: very cold hardy, down to Zone 1

Origin: North American, Europe, Brazil

Why It Works: A Closer Look

Although some fungi have more claim as aphrodisiacs than others, I'm interested in beneficial varieties that can be easily bought or grown. Take the morel, whose aphrodisiac effect comes mostly from its visual stimulation. Morels were originally named *Phallus esculentus* by Carl Linnaeus in 1753. Just one look and you can see where he was going with that. Sadly, the morel was renamed in 1801 to *Morchella esculenta*.

Genus Morchella is derived from *morchel*, an old German word for mushroom, and morel comes from the Latin word *maurus*, meaning brown. And here I was thinking morels were derived from morals... maybe this is why no one consults me for naming plants.

The French writer and mushroom enthusiast Alexandre Dumas praised the morel for its warming effects (much like other aphrodisiacs, i.e., cayenne and cinnamon). This, combined with the high amounts of vitamin D, iron, potassium, and phosphorous, makes morels an excellent way to put some zip into your love life. ✂

GROWING TIPS

Morels, Morchella esculenta, are a member of the Morchellaceae family. The true mushroom "plant" is actually a network of thread-like roots called the mycelium; the fruiting body that we consume appears on the surface after the mycelium has developed below.

Morels live symbiotically on the roots of specific species of trees such as ash, beech, elm, sycamore, cottonwoods, and old apple trees. If you're not a forager you can find morels at the farmers' market – or buy morel spawn from a reputable farmer and grow these mushrooms in your garden at home.

Asparagus and Morels

Serves 6 as a main dish

This robust pairing of two aphrodisiacs, asparagus and morels, is the perfect dish for a young couple in love.

INGREDIENTS

1 pound thick asparagus spears

6-8 ounces fresh morel mushrooms, cleaned and trimmed*

3 tablespoons butter

Salt, to taste

Freshly ground black pepper, to taste

1 tablespoon lemon juice

Snipped fresh chives

Lemon wedges (optional)

Note: If fresh morel mushrooms are not available, substitute 1½ - 2 ounces dried morels. Soak dried mushrooms in warm water for 30 minutes. Drain and pat dry with paper towels.

PREPARATION

Snap off and discard woody bases of asparagus. If desired, scrape off scales. Place a steamer basket in a saucepan. Add water to just below the bottom of the basket, and bring water to boiling. Add asparagus to basket. Cover and reduce heat; steam for 3 - 5 minutes or until crisp-tender. Remove basket; discard liquid.

Meanwhile, in a large skillet, cook morels in 2 tablespoons hot butter over medium heat for 5 minutes, stirring frequently. Season to taste with salt and pepper.

In a large bowl, toss hot asparagus with remaining 1 tablespoon butter and lemon juice to coat. Arrange asparagus and morels on a serving platter and sprinkle with chives. Serve with lemon wedges, if desired.

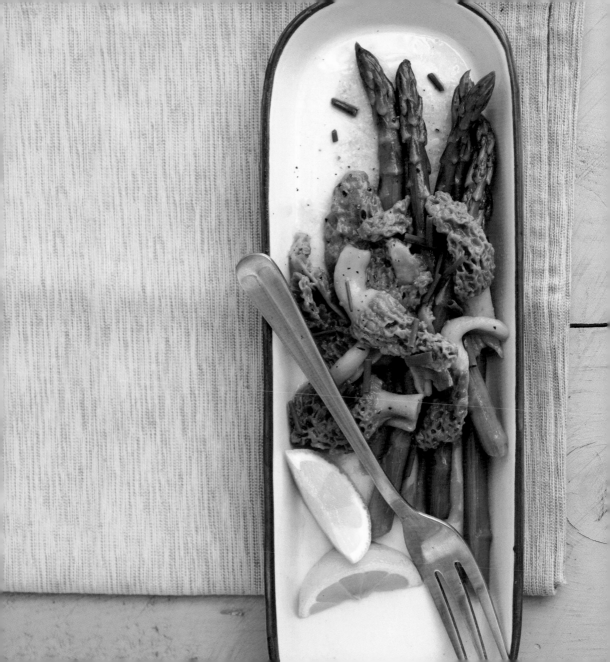

Nutmeg ❧ *Myristica fragrans*

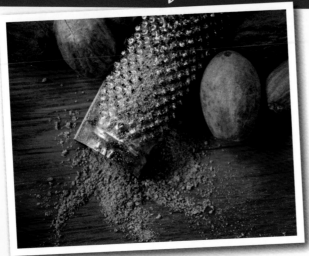

Viagra for women?

COULD IT BE THAT "MOTHER'S LITTLE HELPER" WAS ON THE SPICE RACK ALL along? For centuries in the Middle East, the Orient and Africa, nutmeg has been used as an effective aphrodisiac, and today it is even referred to as "Viagra for women."

In the Middle Ages, nutmeg was used medically for treating ailments from digestive problems to headaches – and even cosmetically to remove freckles. But it's the aphrodisiac benefits that made people sit up straight and reach for the nut and grater.

Nutmeg has been widely used since A.D. 540. In the Middle East, India and China, it was often added to love potions and prescribed by physicians to increase circulation (translation: warm the genital area). Even today in Zanzibar, East Africa, women add nutmeg to their morning porridge on festive days like weddings. It's believed to make women more flirtatious, unusually vivacious, and even giving the feeling of being tipsy, without the alcohol. In India,

NUTMEG

Family: Myristicaceae

Type: Evergreen tree

Color: Brown seed

Harvest Period: Produces fruit year round, but harvest usually occurs in April and November.

Size: 30 to 40 feet high with spreading branches

Soil: Well-drained

Exposure: Sun, part shade

Watering: Moist

pH: 6 to 7

Cold Hardiness Zone: 10

Origin: Spice Islands of Indonesia

---

the spice is used as a stimulant in raising body heat and sweetening breath. A hot body means a "hot" body. No wonder I always feel good after drinking eggnog; and here I always thought it was the warmth of the holidays.

Be careful with this one. Those nuts on your spice rack have a kick to them. Nutmeg is well known in the medical community to be a narcotic. In large doses, it can be hallucinogenic, and too much can

even cause death. Keep your use of nutmeg to eggnog, pies, and a porridge sprinkling for a quick perk up. Malcolm X used nutmeg to get high while in prison when his marijuana stash ran low. You may want to hide it from the kids.

Why It Works: A Closer Look

You don't need a lot. Researchers have found that at low dosages, nutmeg is capable of increasing your libido. Considered a warming herb, a little bit to nutmeg can go a long way. Add nutmeg powder as a flavoring to milk, eggnog, cake and oatmeal. Too much nutmeg can result in toxicity and a hallucinogenic response. Use nutmeg responsibly – limit your use to a pinch.

GROWING TIPS

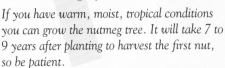

Nutmeg, Myristica fragrans, *is the most well known member of the Myristicaceae family of plants. The nutmeg tree is important for both the nutmeg, which is the actual seed of the tree, and mace, which is the aril (covering) of the seed.*

If you have warm, moist, tropical conditions you can grow the nutmeg tree. It will take 7 to 9 years after planting to harvest the first nut, so be patient.

The Spice Islands, a Far East Eden

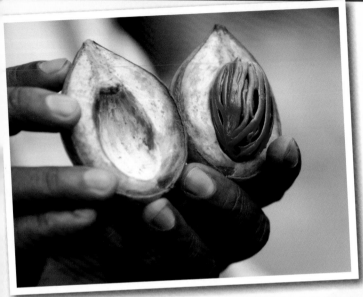

*G*O AHEAD, REACH FOR THE nutmeg to flavor your eggnog or casually insert cloves in the side of your holiday ham. They are just a reach away, right? You actually have quite the commodity sitting on your spice rack. Today, with little money and even less guilt, we have plants with benefits to spice up our daily lives. But it wasn't always that way.

There was a time when cloves and nutmeg (along with mace, the sinuous red aril covering the nutmeg seed, and considered a separate spice), could rival the diamond market of today. Power and destruction, massacres and monopolies – the early spice trade had the makings of a thriller television series, all in the name of a few rare flower parts.

Was the search for these spices because of their aphrodisiac qualities? No, that would play entirely too well into my hands. Instead, I'm competing with the plague. The spices were first imported for their medicinal benefits. The Spice Islands are a small group of islands to the northeast of Indonesia, between Sulawesi and New Guinea. Most commonly referred to as the Banda Islands, they once were the only source of mace, nutmeg, and cloves in the world. In using these spices, Europeans soon learned of their aphrodisiac attributes.

The native Bandanese people had traded peacefully with other nations as early as the Roman Empire. The Chinese, with no plague in sight, certainly benefited from the spices of these tiny islands centuries before the Europeans. Once the Portuguese explorers, like da Gama and Magellan, opened the sea routes around the Cape of Good Hope in the late 15th and early 16th centuries, they laid claim to the spoils of the Spice Islands in the name of Portugal. But it wasn't long before the English and Dutch asserted their own claims. Imagine the new discovery, the desire to possess, the money to be made. As the fortune-hunting lust grew, so did atrocities that progressed to genocide.

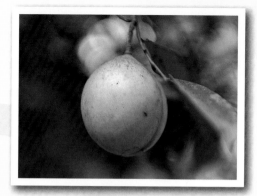

Could the power struggle that caused the ruination of a people have been prevented with some forethought? We're talking about plants and seeds. They can grow in other places, too, couldn't they? This Age of Discovery had also brought explorers to the New World – places with the necessary climate to grow the seeds. In the 18th century, French and Britain entrepreneurs smuggled seeds and seedlings to plant in their own colonial dominions of Mauritius and Grenada (and elsewhere), making these the common spices that they are today. In doing so, monopolies came tumbling down, but not before money was made and empires built. Today the spices sit on our shelves, with most of us unsuspecting of such a checkered past. As an ironic side note, Indonesia, once the sole exporter of cloves, is now a net importer of cloves.

Why the Spice Islands?

Clove and nutmeg trees evolved in isolation on the islands. Why were these spices found only on these Spice Islands? Nobody knows for sure. Certainly, climate and terrain were contributing factors. The Spice Islands are mostly volcanic, covered with lush vegetation in a tropical rainforest climate. Straddling the equator, the islands rise 22,000 feet from the Banda Sea, well suited to growing nutmeg and cloves, among other crops.

As part of the Indonesian "Ring of Fire," the Spice Islands lie along volatile tectonic seams in the Earth's crust. Here, the Eurasian, Pacific and Indo-Australian plates all meet, resulting in frequent earthquakes and volcanic eruptions. These create fertile soils rich in minerals, and together with the tropical rainforest climate, these trees thrive.

Oats ✿ *Avena sativa*

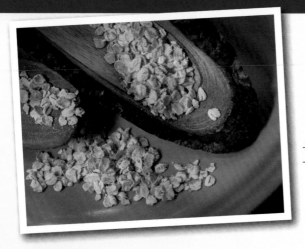

If it's good for horses...

OATS TOOK A WHILE TO CATCH ON. THERE IS EVIDENCE OF OATS BEING cultivated in Bronze Age Switzerland, and in Egypt from 2,000 B.C, but cultivation as a mass food product was slow. For many centuries, oats were used in Chinese medicine as a treatment for low libido, and in the 5th century, the Anglo-Saxons in Britain used oats to treat female infertility.

Oats (*Avena sativa*) were first brought to North America with other grains in 1602 and planted along the coast of Massachusetts. The first oats weren't grown for our oatmeal or even to help with our libidos, but rather for horse feed. However, it was widely known that horses fed oat straw were very energetic.

The oat we have today is probably a mutation of these original wild oats. In a sense, oats are "wild" but that's not where the term "sowing your wild oats" comes from.

Sowing your wild oats. The wild oat, *Avena fatua,* is actually a pernicious weed in the planting fields of Europe. Wild oats were a useless crop since ancient times. The term "sow

OATS

Family: Poaceae

Type: Annual grass

Color: Olive green

Harvest Period: Mid-summer

Size: 4 feet high and 6 inches wide

Soil: Adapts well to most soil types from loam to heavy clay

Exposure: Full sun

Watering: Moist

pH: 6 to 7.5

Cold Hardiness Zone: Annual; grows best in cool weather and tolerates light frost

Origin: Probably the Middle East

---

wild oats" referred to conducting oneself foolishly – to sow weed seed instead of good grain. In 194 B.C., the Roman comic Plautus was the first to use the term.

Why It Works: A Closer Look

All parts of the oat plant are edible and are among the most potent and least expensive libido enhancers available. There is even some science to back it up. Oats have been proven to significantly raise testosterone levels in men. In women, the increase in libido stems from an increase in sexual desire by relaxing the body.

Oatstraw is considered an herbal tonic. It helps bring the nervous system to balance, helps ease anxiety and depression – plus lowering cholesterol and helping with skin conditions. Oats, *Avena sativa*, is an active ingredient in Aveeno® skin care products.

GROWING TIPS

The common oat, Avena sativa, is a member of the Poaceae grass family. Plant it in your garden in the fall as a cover crop for your soil. Oats are one of the easiest and most economical ways to improve your soil, by tilling it back into the ground as "green manure"; but you'll more likely want to grow oats to make a tea.

Making oat tea. *Cut the straw (stalk) of the oat plant into half-inch-sized pieces. Add a few teaspoons in a cup. Add hot water and let steep for 3 to 4 minutes.*

And of course, a bowl of oatmeal in the morning is a great way to start your day.

Sowing Wild Oats Granola

Adapted from a recipe
by Jane Powell

Yield: 5-plus cups

Who knew granola could be so WILD? This crumbled granola mix makes the perfect anytime snack that will have you wanting to sow more and more! The oats, honey, almonds and vanilla are the libido enhancers here.

INGREDIENTS

¼ cup canola oil

¼ cup honey

5 teaspoons vanilla

1 cup dry rolled oats

1 cup raw, hulled sunflower seeds

½ cup wheat germ

½ cup wheat bran

½ cup oat bran

¼ cup flax meal

½ cup sliced almonds

¼ cup pecans

PREPARATION

Preheat oven to 325°F.

Heat the canola oil, honey and vanilla in a saucepan.

Stir together the dry ingredients in a large bowl (or, if you can't find one big enough, several bowls) until everything is well combined.

Pour heated liquid ingredients into the combined dry ingredients. Mix well.

Choose long, wide baking sheets that have sides (the mixture will be thick) and grease them. Spread the mixture into the pans.

Bake for 15 minutes. Remove the pans from the oven, stir the mixture and bake for an additional 15 minutes.

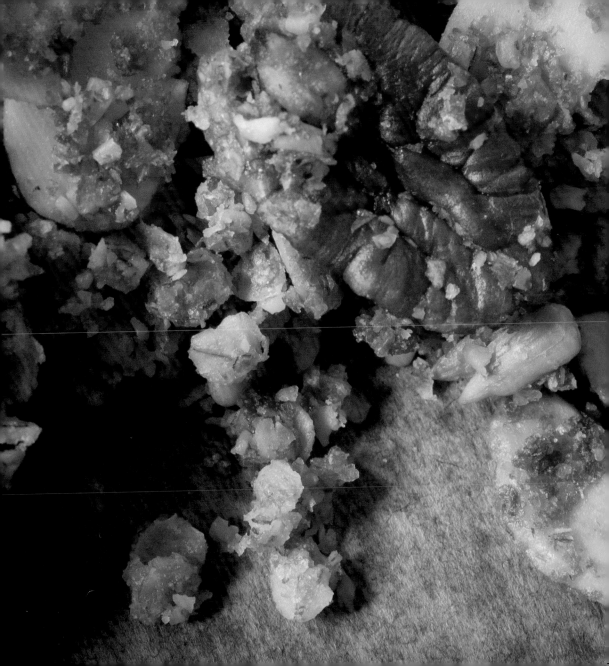

Papaya ❧ *Carica papaya*

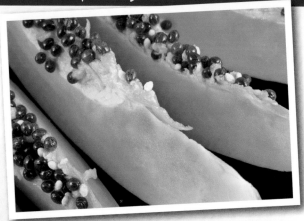

Don't ask for it in Cuba

I SEE PAPAYA AT THE GROCERY STORE AND THINK IT WOULD BE FUN TO EAT, but then I never know what to do with it! With a hard, fleshy skin, some are large and others are small by comparison, with color choices of green or yellow. Unfortunately for me, growing up in Middle America didn't offer many opportunities to go out and pick this exotic fruit for an afternoon snack.

When I cracked open a papaya recently, my heart pitter-pattered at the sight of all those seeds. I blushed. It was shockingly sexy, for some reason. (Note: I'm in the P's; well entrenched in aphrodisiacs.)

Papayas have long been revered by the Latin American Indians. Discovering papaya in the Americas, the Spanish and Portuguese introduced it to other tropical and subtropical lands, such as India, the Philippines, and parts of Africa. It caught on fast. Papaya is definitely a fun, sexy fruit. Even today, Guatemalan men eat papayas as an aphrodisiac. And beware of saying how much you like papaya when you're in Cuba. Papaya is a Cuban slang word for vagina.

PAPAYA

Family: Caricaceae

Type: Broadleaf evergreen

Color: Green, with yellowish-white blooms

Harvest Period: Bears fruit throughout the year

Size: 6 to 20 feet high and 3 to 15 feet wide

Soil: Well-drained loamy soil

Exposure: Full sun

Watering: Medium

pH: 6 to 7

Cold Hardiness Zone: 10

Origin: Central America

An anti-aphrodisiac, too? For the men, make sure your fruit is ripe before you eat it, because some will argue that an unripened papaya will reduce your sexual desire. So unless that is your intention, eat your fruit ripe. If you are shipwrecked on a lonely island, go for the green, unripened fruit. You'll thank me later.

Why It Works: A Closer Look

Papaya is estrogenic, mimicking compounds that act as the hormone estrogen, and stimulating the female libido. It is also rich in vitamins A, B, C, E and K, with antioxidants such as carotenes, flavonoids. As an added bonus, papaya contains the minerals potassium and magnesium, making it a well-balanced fruit for a healthy heart – and good for blood flow.

GROWING TIPS

Papaya, Carica papaya is a member of the Caricaceae family of flowering plants with only six genera and about 35 species. You are not likely to be able to grow papaya at home unless you live in a tropical or subtropical region,. This fruit is intolerant of frost, preferring a warmer climate. You could grow papaya as a container plant and overwinter indoors, though. It makes a nice ornamental houseplant tree.

The flowers of the papaya plant are fragrant and trumpet-shaped, and bloom throughout the year. The male flowers have long racemes; the female flowers form in small clusters or are solitary, and give way to a smooth-skinned green fruit that ripens to yellow-orange. Oh, and the peppery-tasting seeds are edible.

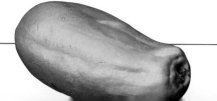

Parsley 🌿 *Petroselinum crispum*

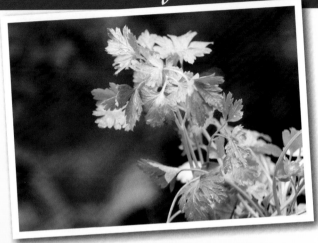

A healthier, friskier you

AT THE RISK OF ALARMING, I HAVE TO TELL YOU THAT PARSLEY WAS LONG associated with death. According to Greek lore, parsley sprouted from the spilled blood of Archemorus, the old fertility king, whose name means "forerunner of death." What sprouted could have been what's called, fool's parsley, *Aethusa cynapium*, thus giving actual parsley, *Petroselinum crispum*, a bad rap for many a year. I can understand that if they grew side-by-side in nature, and they looked so much alike, it would be smart to stay away from both.

Through the centuries, the Greeks, Romans, and Christians as well, associated parsley with death. Wreaths of parsley were laid on Greek tombs, Romans dedicated the herb to Persephone (who lived 6 months of the year in the Underworld) and used it in funeral rites. And early Christians consecrated parsley to Saint Peter, guardian of the gates of heaven.

A fork in the road. Somewhere along the way, the subtle differences between fool's parsley and actual parsley were determined, and the high value of parsley realized. Parsley began

PARSLEY

Family: Apiacea (or Umbelliferae)

Type: Biennial, suitable as an annual

Color: Green

Harvest Period: Anytime; snip as needed

Size: 0.75 to 1 foot high and wide

Soil: Most soil types

Exposure: Full sun to part shade

Watering: Medium

pH: 6 to 7

Cold Hardiness Zone: 2 to 11

Origin: Europe and the Mediterranean

to be widely appreciated for its medicinal, culinary – and yes, aphrodisiac properties.

Why It Works: A Closer Look

I would class parsley as one of the milder aphrodisiacs. Not dramatic, but a valuable plant to have in your potager, nonetheless. When we consider the many ways a plant with benefits can do its job, we often find a number of elements working together to smooth the way to enjoyable sex, simply

by removing impediments. The benefits of parsley are in the roots, seeds, and leaves. Its leaves make a superb breath freshener, for starters. Parsley's antibacterial action will keep the body sweeter. The plant is a powerhouse of important vitamins and minerals that aid the immune system and benefit the liver, spleen, digestive, and endocrine systems. It is commonly used to combat urinary track infections and prostate conditions. The root is also high in estrogen-like hormones and is thought to aid in menstrual and PMS distress. All of which can lead to a healthier, friskier you. ✀

GROWING TIPS

Parsley, Petroselinum crispum, *is a biennial herb in the* Apiacea *(or* Umbelliferae*) family, commonly known as the carrot or parsley family. Easy to grow, parsley will tolerate a wide range of soils and sun exposure. There are three kinds of parsley: curly leaved* (P. crispum), *the most popular in culinary use and as a bedding plant; Italian or flat-leaved* (P. neapolitanum), *stronger flavored; and Hamburg* (P. tuberosum), *grown for its parsnip-like roots. Parsley makes a great container plant for the patio, deck, window boxes, or balcony.*

Passionflower ❧ *Passiflora incarnata*

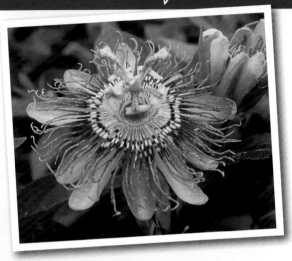

A Peruvian delight

IN MY HUMBLE OPINION, THE PASSIONFLOWER *(PASSIFLORA INCARNATA)* IS ONE of the most beautiful flowers in the world. When friends visit and see these blooms for the first time, their faces brighten with wonder. Fascination is the word that comes to mind.

Passion is as Peruvians do. The *passion* in passionflower would normally suggest romance, but it is actually derived from the Passion of Christ. According to legend, a Jesuit priest in the early 1600s discovered the vine growing wild in Peru. In a vision that evening, the priest associated each part of the flower– from its petals to its anthers – with the Passion of Christ. As a perhaps ironic counterpoint, the Peruvians enjoyed the flower for its aphrodisiac benefits.

The Aztecs used passionflower as a pain reliever and sedative to ease muscle tension and calm the mind. The Native Americans taught the early European settlers the many benefits of the passionflower's roots and leaves. Passionflower's effectiveness in treating a host of issues

PASSIONFLOWER

Family: Passifloraceae

Type: Deciduous Vine

Color: Purples

Harvest Period: July to September

Size: 6 to 8 feet high; 3 to 6 feet wide

Soil: Well-drained soil

Exposure: Full sun to part shade

Watering: Medium, tolerates drought

pH: 6.1 to 7.5

Cold Hardiness Zone: 5 to 9

Origin: The Americas

that trouble the human body and mind – like headaches and seizures, insomnia and anxiety – has long been known; but it is only recently that scientific evidence began to support what we're here today to consider: its aphrodisiac properties.

Why It Works: A Closer Look

Passionflower (*Passiflora incarnate*) contains chrysin, a bioflavonoid that encourages a higher rate of testosterone, perfect for body builders…and (naturally) guys who need a little boost in their lovin'. Chrysin has also been proven to reduce stress and performance anxiety. Recent studies in benzoflavone moiety (BZF), another component of passionflower, show the plant's potential in counteracting the effects of aging on male sexuality. Granted, these studies were performed on male rats, who had their sexual vigor restored – but all science has to start somewhere! ✀

GROWING TIPS

The passionflower (Passiflora incarnata) is in the Passifloraceae family. The fruit of the passionflower, also known as May-pops, can be eaten fresh off the vine or made into jelly. The passionflower, is a vigorous grower, so you may need to keep an eye on it and give it plenty of space. A native to the Americas, passionflower vine can be found growing in Eastern North America and south to Florida and Texas.

The passionflower vine is also the host plant for many butterflies such as the Gulf fritillary, the Zebra Heliconians, and the Crimson patch (Chlosyne janais).

Grow in full sun to part shade with average, medium moisture, and well-drained soil. A worthy addition to any garden that can grow it, it will catch the eye of anyone who comes by to admire your flower bed!

Pine Nut ❧ *Pinus pinea*

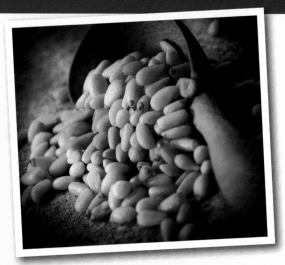

Take 100 at bedtime and call me in the morning

𝒯HE ANCIENT PEOPLE OF THE MEDITERRANEAN WERE WILD ABOUT THE PINE nut, where it has been known as an aphrodisiac since the first nut was popped in the mouth of an unsuspecting lad.

Harvested from the pine tree, *Pinus pinea,* pine nuts have been cultivated for over 6,000 years. The taste is very pleasing and complements many dishes, particularly pasta with basil pesto (see pesto recipe on page 22). Poets and physicians alike have suggested pine nuts for use in love potions. In at least one case, the nut came with a warning of its sexual enhancing powers when, in 2 A.D., the Roman poet Ovid pointed to the pine nut (among others on a list of aphrodisiacs) in his poem *Ars amatoria* (The Art of Love), challenging the serious moral reform efforts of Augustus. Marcus Guavas Apicius, a Roman gourmet (1st century A.D.) – whose recipes were used up through the Middle Ages – recommended a mixture of pine nuts, cooked onions, white mustard, and pepper to achieve lustful love.

PINE NUTS

Family: Pinaceae

Type: Needled evergreen; conifer

Color: Green (tree), creamy white (nuts)

Harvest Period: Fall

Size: 40 to 60 Feet high and 20 to 40 feet wide.

Soil: Moist, well-drained soils, but not waterlogged. Drought tolerant

Exposure: Full sun

Watering: Dry to medium

pH: Tolerant of most pH soil

Cold Hardiness Zone: 8 to 10

Origin: Mediterranean region (Southern Europe to Turkey and Lebanon) and parts of northern Africa

---

Prescription for pleasure. In the 2nd century, the famed physician Galen prescribed to his patients a mixture of pine seeds, honey and almonds, to be taken before bedtime for three consecutive evenings to increase sexual intimacy. We find the same prescription in the 15th century Arabic love manual, *The Perfumed Garden of Sensual Delights*, where Sheikh Nefzawi advises that a man should eat 20 almonds and 100 pine nuts, along with a glassful of thick honey, for three nights before bedtime. All three are in my book, too. How affirming that Galen and the good sheikh agree with my selections!

Why It Works: A Closer Look

Let's get to the point: pine nuts are high in energizing zinc, which is essential for the production of testosterone, thus increasing the sex drive for both men and women. Like most nuts, pine nuts also offer cardiovascular benefits and are a good source of thiamin, iron, magnesium, and manganese. You want to have those cardiovascular benefits to keep the blood flowing well. Need I say more? ✀

GROWING TIPS

Pinus pinea prefers moist, sandy, well-drained soils. It tolerates most soil pH. In the Pinaceae family, pine nut trees grow best in cooler climates with dry summers.

True pines don't make good indoor houseplants, but Pinus pinea are often sold as indoor Christmas trees during the holidays. In warmer climates, zones 8 - 10, they can be planted outdoors after the holidays.

Warm Quinoa Salad

From the kitchen of
Carolyn Binder,
Cowlick Cottage Farm

Serves 6

Quinoa: can you say "KEEN-WAH?" In doing so, it will be the beginning of a long, tasteful relationship. High in protein, this gluten free, fiber-rich grain goes well with most anything, but Carolyn paired it nicely with pine nuts, shrimp (both aphrodisiacs), roasted broccoli and feta – putting this bodacious dish on the O-list.

INGREDIENTS

3 cups cooked quinoa

I head fresh broccoli, cut into small florets and stems

I onion, sliced thin

3 garlic cloves, peeled and sliced thin

²/₃ cup pine nuts

Salt and pepper, to taste

¼ cup olive oil

I pound langoustines, precooked and thawed, if frozen (or substitute shrimp)

A squeeze of fresh lemon juice

½ cup Feta cheese, crumbled

PREPARATION

Preheat oven to 400°F.
Prepare the quinoa according to package directions. At the same time, toss the broccoli with the onion, garlic, pine nuts and olive oil in a roasting pan, making sure that everything is coated with the oil. Season to taste with salt and pepper. Roast in the oven for 15-20 minutes, tossing occasionally, until the edges of the broccoli start to crisp and the pine nuts are golden.

Turn the warm quinoa onto a serving platter and top with the broccoli mixture.

Top with the langoustines, a squeeze of fresh lemon juice, Feta cheese and an extra drizzle of the olive oil.

Serve and enjoy!

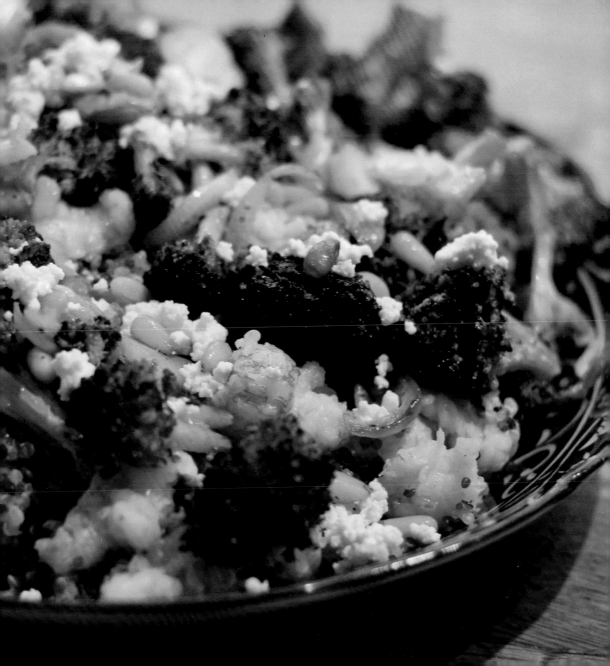

Pomegranate · *Punica granatum*

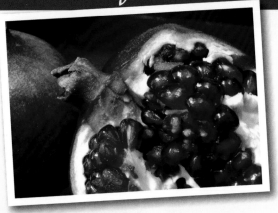

The color of desire

$\mathcal{I}$F YOU LOOK DEEP INTO THE LORE OF CULTURES WHERE THE POMEGRANATE grows – as far back as 4,000 B.C. – you will see it revered as a symbol of fertility, rebirth, and health. This sensual and unusual fruit can be found at the center of many a love legend. Its obvious benefits arise from its appearance, scent, texture, and taste, but its chemical gifts work unseen to heighten arousal.

Just cut one open. It's easy to see just how sexy this fruit is and why ancient cultures associated it with desire and seduction.

In Greek mythology, the pomegranate played a crucial role in the seduction of Persephone by Hades, god of the Underworld. To keep her from returning to the world of light, he offered her pomegranate seeds to eat, knowing that by eating them she would have to stay with him. In a deal made with her mother, Demeter, she was allowed to leave the Underworld for half of each year. The fruit was also the symbol of Dionysian rites (celebrated with sexual abandon), and was a culinary symbol of Aphrodite.

In China, candied pomegranate seeds were served at weddings to ensure fertility. And the *Kama Sutra*, you say? This traditional text on the finer points of lovemaking specifically

POMEGRANATE

Family: Lythraceae

Type: Deciduous shrub

Color: Vibrant scarlet red to orange (sometimes white or variegated) bloom and red-orange fruit

Harvest Period: Fall

Size: 6 to 20 feet high and 4 to 15 feet wide

Soil: Well-drained soil

Exposure: Full sun

Watering: Dry to medium

pH: 5.5 to 7

Cold Hardiness Zone: 8 to 11

Origin: Eastern Mediterranean to Himalayas

suggests the pomegranate and offers recipes said to both amplify desire and enhance physical pleasure.

In Persian Christianity, the fruit Eve plucked from the Tree of Knowledge and shared with Adam was not an apple, but a pomegranate. You'll see it as a frequent symbol in Christianity, representing hope, eternal life, and the Church itself. Thus, for Persian Christians, the pomegranate becomes both the forbidden and celebrated fruit.

Why It Works: A Closer Look

Pomegranate is one of the super fruits, contributing to a healthy body and all that that implies. It's packed with micronutrients such as polyphenols (specifically, tannins and flavonoids, which are known to increase female libido) and zinc (critical for a man's sexual performance). Rich in antioxidants, pomegranate provides B vitamins (thiamine, riboflavin, niacin, B5, B6 and folate), vitamin C, dietary fiber, magnesium, phosphorus, and potassium. An all-round plant with benefits.

GROWING TIPS

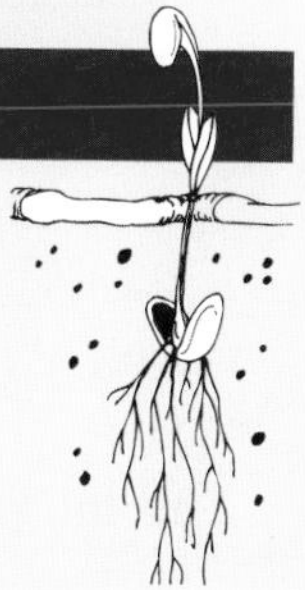

The pomegranate, Punica granatum, *is a member of the Lythraceae family.*

The deciduous shrub can be grown as a tree in the home garden; compact varieties like the 3-foot-tall 'Nana,' which will fit almost any size garden, even a balcony, and can be grown as an indoor plant when placed in front of a sunny window. The fruit is proportional to the size of the plant.

Add pomegranate seed to your salads and rice dishes or blend into a juice for a refreshing treat.

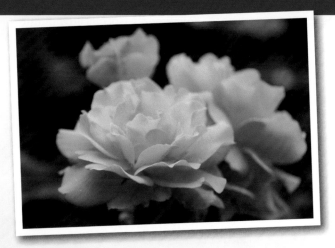

From innocence to passion

ROSES ARE THE UNIVERSAL DOOR KNOCKER TO THE HEART. WE RECEIVE ROSES when we succeed, we give roses when we apologize, not to mention birthdays, anniversaries, Mother's Day… the list goes on. For sweet memories we plant roses in a garden and press petals between the pages of a special album.

The language of flowers. These fragrant flowers have been part of our mythology and lore for thousands of years. The color of a rose speaks a language all its own. In Greek mythology, the goddess of love, Aphrodite, was born from dripping sea foam that transformed into white roses, symbolizing purity and innocent love. When Aphrodite was older and rushed to the aid of her wounded and dying lover Adonis, however, she pricked her foot on a white rose bush, whereupon the roses turned red from her blood. From purity to desire; from innocence to passion.

Over time, other colors spoke to us as well: yellow to convey warm feelings and contentment, pink to express joyfulness. We can't help inviting roses into our hearts. Rose water, rose

ROSE

Family: Rosaceae

Type: Floribunda rose

Color: Apricot

Harvest Period: Seasonal, repeat bloomer

Size: 3 feet high and wide

Soil: Organically rich, well-drained

Exposure: Full sun

Watering: Medium

pH: Slightly acidic at 6.5

Cold Hardiness Zone: 6 to 10

Origin: USA Pat. 16250

petals, and rose-scented oils have long been used in sherbets and pastries, sipped as tea, and made into sachets for scenting apparel. There's no escaping our attraction to this delicate and lovely flower.

Just what is it about roses?

Why It Works: A Closer Look

While the act of receiving roses itself can be an arousal stimulus, there are other aphrodisiac qualities at work. The mere aroma of roses or rose water stimulates the sensations and relaxes the mind, thanks to the neurotransmitter phenylethylamine, sometimes called "the love chemical" for the euphoric feelings it creates.

Feeling like some rose petal tea right now? Simply pour 3/4 cup of boiling water over a pinch of rose petals and let steep. Ahhh... ✂

GROWING TIPS

It would be silly of me to suggest one rose to grow out of the entire Rosaceae family that includes 2830 species in 95 genera. Yet I did. Meet Rosa 'Honey Perfume.'

A floribunda, 'Honey Perfume' has a delicately sweet scent, with apricot flowers on multi-branches. I think floribundas are sexier than a tall, single-stemmed rose. For me, the ultimate expression of love is a bouquet of roses cut from my own garden. Since roses are not blooming in most of our gardens in February, though, might I suggest wooing your beloved on Valentine's Day with a box of chocolates, a rose catalogue, and a note saying you will plant and maintain the chosen rose bush? And don't forget to use a natural, organic fertilizer called Moo Poo tea. Despite the unromantic name, it really does wonders for roses.

Saffron ❧ *Crocus sativus*

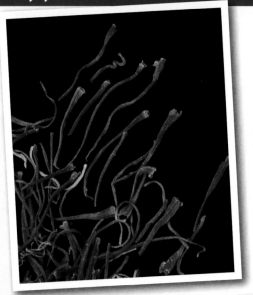

The world's most expensive sexy spice

𝓗IGHLY PRAISED IN CLASSICAL GREECE FOR ITS COLORING AND AROMATIC properties, saffron has long been used in a variety of ways, culinary and otherwise – as a help for insomnia and even as a cure for hangovers caused by wine. But it's the aphrodisiac reputation of this crocus spice that has my attention. Imagine the luxurious life of Cleopatra, the last pharaoh of Egypt – a woman known for her brilliance and for her secrets of seduction. It is said that before she had an important tryst she bathed in the stigma (saffron threads) of the crocus plant, in expectation of the aphrodisiac effects.

Saffron is the crimson red, protruding stigma of *Crocus sativus* – the female reproductive system and pollen collector of this flowering bulb. It takes up to 75,000 crocus blossoms to produce a pound of saffron spice. Because of this, saffron has long been the world's most expensive

SAFFRON

Family: Iridaceae

Type: Flowering bulb (corm)

Color: Lavender purple

Harvest Period: Fall

Size: 0.25 to 0.5 feet high and wide

Soil: Well-drained

Exposure: Full sun to part shade

Watering: Medium

pH: 6 to 8

Cold Hardiness Zone: 3 to 8

Origin: Mediterranean region

spice. Luckily, it only takes two or three threads to flavor your rice or stir-fry. Eastern cultures mix saffron in milk and in desserts for flavor – and for its reputed aphrodisiac benefits.

During the early Renaissance, saffron was worth its weight in gold. Naturally, corruption ensued, with substitutes and resulting adulterations, to the point that King Henry VIII condemned to death any adulterers of his cherished spice.

Too much of a good thing? There is disagreement about whether saffron is toxic or actually a detoxifier, but to be safe, one should not consume extravagantly large amounts of this aromatic plant part (if you can afford it)... Death by saffron?

Why It Works: A Closer Look

There is certainly anecdotal evidence of saffron as an aphrodisiac, although Western science attributes it to the placebo effect. But a 2008 study conducted on male rats (stay with me here) at the Mashhad University of Medical Science in Iran found that rats that ingested saffron had increased sex drive. Saffron contains crocin, a natural carotenoid chemical shown to have aphrodisiac properties. I'm willing to take the leap of faith that it works on human males as well. ✀

GROWING TIPS

For something so expensive, Crocus sativus *is easy to grow in the home garden, providing the spice as close as your front steps. In the Iridaceae family, along with the genus Iris, saffron can be harvested with tweezers, dried and stored in an air-tight container. Saffron grows best in areas with a long, dry summer. Plant in a gravely area, like a rock garden, for increased success.*

Sage ❦ *Salvia officinalis 'Tricolor'*

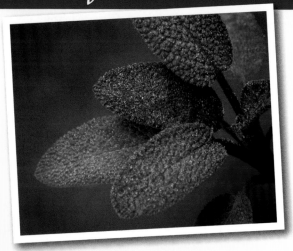

Stimulating to the touch

𝒥UST THE SOUND OF THE WORD SAGE FEELS SERIOUS AND IMPORTANT. Sage, as in "sage advice," is associated with wisdom. What if we could simply grow wisdom in our gardens? How easy life would be.

Sage was cultivated by the ancient Greeks, Romans and Egyptians. A plant that grows widely and without care, sage has long been used for cooking and medicine, and in certain ceremonial practices. Its aphrodisiac qualities haven't always been its principal charms, but we'll talk about those in a moment. The Greeks consumed sage to bring wisdom as well as to gain long life – and possibly even immortality. The idea being that since sage is such a long-lived perennial, its powers could also be possessed by the gardener who grows it.

If you were a young Roman couple, sage would hang on your bedpost as a help with domestic virtue (whatever that might imply, beyond simple fidelity). In Native American cultures sage is a sacred herb used ceremonially as a smudge. As the smoke from the smudge rises, it

SAGE

Family: Lamiaceae

Type: Herbaceous perennial

Color: Tricolor - green, white and purple

Harvest Period:

Size: 1 to 1.5 feet high and wide

Soil: Most types

Exposure: Full sun

Watering: Dry to medium

pH: 4.5 to 8

Cold Hardiness Zone: 6 to 9, suitable as an annual

Origin: Mediterranean and northern Africa

---

carries prayers to the Great Spirit. In feng shui, sage is a purifier of energies in a space.

Let's be direct. Sage can also be placed directly on the skin for a stimulating effect. Add sage to your bath water for similar invigorating results.

Why It Works: A Closer Look

Compared to other aphrodisiacs, sage is weak but plentiful, and that makes up for its shortcomings. Sage could easily be growing off your back deck. You never know when you might need a quick fix.

Sage's stimulating benefit comes from the presence of estrogen, phenolic acids and flavonoids – qualifying this herb as an aphrodisiac, albeit a bit more subtle than many. Try drinking sage tea by pouring eight ounces of boiling water over about ten large, fresh sage leaves. Steep for five minutes and strain. You may find the taste bitter, so add honey for sweetness. ✂

GROWING TIPS

Sage, Salvia officinalis *'Tricolor', is a member of the mint family Lamiaceae. Most members of the Lamiaceae family of plants are characterized by square stems and opposite leaves. If you've never felt the stems of a member of the mint family, do! It's interesting to feel the difference between these stems and those with a cylindrical shape.*

Grow in full sun, with average to medium moisture. Wet soils are fatal to sage.

The ancient Greeks, Romans and Egyptians grew the straight species, Salvia officinalis, but the new selection 'Tricolor' would also be a welcome addition to the home garden.

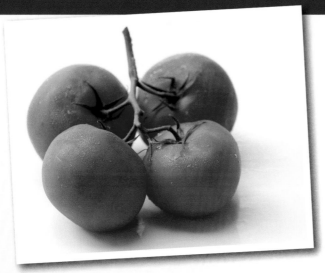

The sinfully suggestive love apple

CONSIDERING THAT TOMATOES WERE ONCE ASSOCIATED WITH THE DEVIL, one has to wonder how they became a symbol of love and sensuality. Or maybe you just have to look at one to get the idea. The tomato grew only in Mesoamerica until the Spanish Conquistadors brought it back to Europe in the early 16th century. The Church saw the red, sexy, plump tomatoes and quickly dubbed them the devil's fruit, a sinful indulgence. There may be some truth to the tomato's sinfulness, though, if you're moved by its seductive harlot-red color and smooth, sensuous flesh… Scandalous! Forbidden! Pass the salt, please.

What's in a name? It was the French who referred to the tomato as *pomme d'amour*, or love apple. Ahh, the French, elevating anything and everything to love! Some spoilsports believe *pomme d'amour* was actually a corruption of a Spanish phrase meaning apple of the Moors. Poor unromantic souls.

TOMATO

Family: Solanaceae

Type: Annual, indeterminate vine

Color: Green leaves, yellow flowers, red fruit

Harvest Period: Summer

Size: 6 to 8 feet

Soil: loamy, fertile soil

Exposure: Full sun

Watering: Medium

pH: 5.5 to 7.5

Cold Hardiness Zone: Above freezing

Origin: South America

The tomato was considered poisonous at one time, possibly due to its membership in the nightshade family and being mistaken for the deadly nightshade plant. While tomato's leaves are indeed toxic, its rich meat is quite the opposite. Either way, I'm with the French.

Why It Works: A Closer Look

The beautiful, elegant, shapely, lusty tomato made the list on looks alone. There is no strong folklore or science to confirm its aphrodisiac benefits. But don't underestimate the power of suggestion. As I wrote in the Introduction: just thinking that something is an aphrodisiac is enough to make it work as one. In my own version of the Doctrine of Signatures, that bright red color and those smooth curves are an obvious prescription for arousal. ✀

GROWING TIPS

The tomato is one of the most important cultivated members of the Solanaceae clan, otherwise known as the deadly nightshade family. Also on the family tree are the potato, the eggplant, tobacco and petunias. The Solanaceae family consists of 2,500 species of flowering plants in 102 genera and can be found worldwide, but they are most abundant in tropical Latin America.

There are dozens of varieties of tomatoes, the most common being the all-purpose globe tomatoes that you can eat raw or cooked. Plum tomatoes (aka Italian or Roma) are perfect for a delicious red sauce, and bite-size cherry and cocktail types are ideal for snacking and salads.

The deep red Campari (shown here) is a type of large cocktail tomato noted for its juiciness, high sugar level and low acidity. In the grocery store, they are often presented in clusters still clinging on the vine.

Tomato Temptation

Serves 4-6 as a main dish,
8 as a side dish

Tomato Temptation is one of my husband's favorite dishes, so it is also mine [wink]. Tomatoes are one sexy fruit; and coupling the red orb with feta, Italian dressing, cannelloni beans and rustic bread forms the building blocks of a special relationship – if for no other reason than the beauty of this freshly-prepared dish.

INGREDIENTS

5-6 tomatoes (It's fun to use different colors and varieties)

1 cup cannelloni beans (optional)

½ cup Italian salad dressing (can be light)

1½ cups feta cheese, crumbled

4 – 5 half-inch-thick slices of rustic bread

pepper, to taste

PREPARATION

Dice tomatoes into about ½-inch pieces and place in a bowl. Add cannelloni beans, if desired. Mix with Italian dressing and top with feta cheese.

Toast the bread and tear it into ½-inch pieces. Add to the tomato salad and mix in just before serving. Add pepper, to taste, if desired.

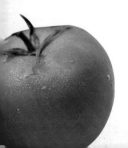

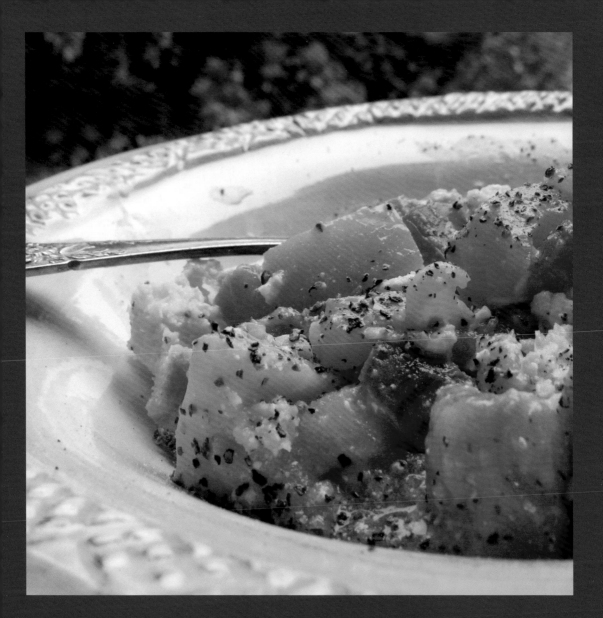

Vanilla ❧ *Vanilla planifolia*

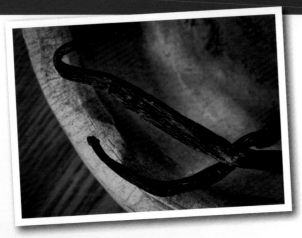

Can you guess what it does to men?

*V*ANILLA IS AN ORCHID! WHAT A FITTING PLANT WITH BENEFITS: SENSUAL, SEXY, and satisfying to receive. There are about 26,000 orchids, but the *Vanilla planifolia* is the only one that is edible. The vanilla we pay so dearly for is actually a pod produced by the flower.

The ancient Totonac Indians of Mexico believed vanilla to be an aphrodisiac. This notion probably stemmed from the Totonac myth about Princess Xanat. She was in love with a mortal man but forbidden to marry him because of her divine nature. When she and her lover fled to the forest, they were captured and beheaded; an orchid grew from the spot where their blood touched the ground.

When vanilla was introduced to Europe, its pods quickly became prized as an aphrodisiac – the belief being that vanilla could transform an ordinary man into an astonishing lover. No doubt they had heard about Montezuma's great, ahem, appetites.

Vanilla chocolate a la Conquistador. The ancient Aztecs mixed vanilla with chocolate to make a potent aphrodisiac drink. Montezuma didn't miss a chance to double his aphrodisiac

VANILLA

Family: Orchidaceae

Type: Evergreen orchid vine

Color: Brown pods when the vanilla bean dries

Harvest Period: At maturity, about six months after flowering

Size: 50 to 60 feet high and 4 to 6 feet wide

Soil: Light mix

Exposure: Part shade to full shade

Watering: Medium

pH: 6.6 to 7.5

Cold Hardiness Zone: 11 to 12

Origin: Florida, West Indies, Central and South America

pleasure! (See Chocolate, page 38.) It was also an immediate hit with the Spanish Conquistador Hernan Cortes, who, we hear, drank the concoction after his New World conquests in 1518.

By the way, Montezuma got his revenge: once Cortes introduced vanilla to Spain, it took 300 years before anyone could figure out how to propagate the flower. Only a certain Mexican hummingbird or a Melipona bee could do this naturally.

Why It Works: A Closer Look

The aphrodisiac qualities are believed to come from the scent and flavor of the vanilla seedpod – with particular benefit arising when paired with chocolate. To add a little recent science to the lore, when neurologist Alan Hirsch of the Smell & Taste Treatment and Research Foundation conducted controlled tests to see which fragrance combinations increased penile blood flow, guess which scent aroused men the very most: vanilla.

GROWING TIPS

Vanilla, Vanilla planifolia, hails mostly from Mexico. If you live in a climate lucky enough to grow it, please do. A good vine can produce 100 pods per year. Vanilla comes in two varieties: a plain and a variegated form. If you are able to grow it but are outside the native range, you will have to hand-pollinate in order to produce fruit (since you won't have the native Melipona bee to do the work for you). These black beans develop over a period of eight to nine months and grow eight inches long.

Walnut ❧ *Juglans nigra*

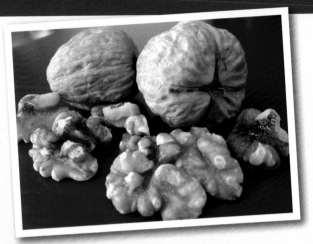

The super nut

MOST OF US DON'T GIVE MUCH THOUGHT TO THE BLACK WALNUT. SURE, WE find them sitting in a nut bowl during Thanksgiving or hanging in brightly colored packaging at the grocery store, ready to flavor a recipe. But is there a hidden benefit here – something earthy and arousing, especially for men? Could be. Walnuts have been around since the Neolithic Age (about 8,000 BC), expanding throughout Europe sometime between 6,000 and 2,000 BC. The black walnut might very well have been the aphrodisiac that kept civilization growing, and growing strong.

Word gets around. The ancient Greeks and Persians were the first to cultivate black walnuts and link them to love and fertility. The Romans eventually caught wind and took a liking to them; whole black walnuts have been found in the ruins of Pompeii.

The Romans associated the walnut with the Juno, goddess of women and marriage. The ancients were so smitten with the fertility power of walnuts that wedding guests would throw them at the bride and groom. Some things do change for the better.

WALNUT

Family: Juglandaceae

Type: Deciduous tree

Color: Light brown nuts

Harvest Period: Fall

Size: 75 to 100 feet high and wide

Soil: Rich, well-drained soil

Exposure: Full sun

Watering: Medium

pH: 5 to 8

Cold Hardiness Zone: 4 to 9

Origin: Eastern United States

Farther north, in Medieval times and later, we hear of French peasants in the countryside who believed the walnut tree possessed aphrodisiac powers. When an object of a young man's affections wasn't looking, he would try to sneak a leaf of the tree into her shoe. An awkward way to woo, but not as painful as flinging walnuts at her.

Why It Works: A Closer Look

Today, there are so many studies on the health value of the walnut that its use as an aphrodisiac is almost overshadowed. Rest assured, there's merit to the claim. Black walnuts contain arginine, an amino acid that's absorbed and transformed in the body to make nitric oxide, which enlarges blood vessels and enhances blood flow to the penis. There is even a company out there that produces a walnut-based Viagra replacement. Good luck with that.

Walnuts are considered a super food because they contain omega-3 fatty acids, B vitamins, vitamin E and folic acid, as well as an abundance of highly beneficial minerals, such as calcium, iron, magnesium, potassium, and zinc.

GROWING TIPS

Black walnut Juglans nigra is a monster of a tree, but it would be pretty awesome to have one (if you have land to support it). A member of the Juglandaceae family, black walnut prefers moist, organically-rich, well-drained soil in full sun.

Black walnut trees secrete juglone (from both leaves and roots) in the soil, a poisonous substance that keeps other plants from growing under and near the tree. Juglone has a particularly negative effect on fruit trees. It's best to grow black walnut in relative isolation from other plants.

Watermelon ❧ *Citrullus lanatus*

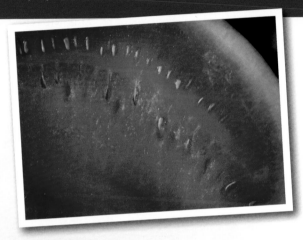

The fruit of multiple pleasures

*A*HH, WATERMELON. WHAT OTHER FRUIT RELAXES YOU TO THE POINT WHERE eating outside is actually preferred? Outside, you can let the sweet watermelon run down your chin, onto your shirt and into your lap. Not to mention spitting those shiny black seeds wherever you want.

Watermelon wasn't always fun and games. In older cultures it was a valuable source of water for desert travel and living. Somewhere along the way, someone must have gotten hungry enough to eat the seeds and the rind, though – and things began to happen. In aphrodisiac terms, the rind is the business end of the fruit.

You either love it or – love it! Watermelon was enjoyed in every part of the world where it was traded. From its African origins, it spread to India in 800 A.D. and China in 1,100 A.D., where the seeds were eaten and crushed for their edible oils. From the Mediterranean trade routes into Europe, it reached the New World, where it flourished. Florida was producing watermelons by 1576. In the late 19th century, Mark Twain wrote in his book *Puddn'head Wilson:* "The true southern watermelon is a boon apart and not to be men-

WATERMELON

Family: Cucuribitaceae

Type: Annual vine

Color: Green

Harvest Period: End of summer

Size: 0.75 to 1.5 feet high and 10 to 15 feet wide

Soil: Fertile loam

Exposure: Full sun

Watering: Medium

pH: 6 to 6.8

Cold Hardiness Zone: 2 to 11, annual

Origin: Africa

rind. The inner white rind contains citrulline, an amino acid that not only benefits the cardiovascular and immune systems, but also enables the body to relax and expand blood vessels, thus facilitating the libido.

Studies suggest you have to eat a lot of rind to get the effects of citrulline, so juice the rind with the fruit or reach for a jar of pickled watermelon rinds for a quick aphrodisiac snack. Just be careful with the green part, which can cause stomachaches and cramps – anything but romantic! ✀

tioned with commoner things. It is chief of this world's luxuries, king by the grace of God over all the fruits of the earth. When one has tasted it, he knows what the angels eat." Pretty high praise for this sweet, delectable fruit! I wonder if the praise is also for the rind. Hmm.

Why It Works: A Closer Look

To get to the aphrodisiac components of watermelon, one must go beyond the fruit's red richness and deep into the layers of the

GROWING TIPS

Watermelon, Citrullus lanatus, is a member of the Cucuribitaceae family. This important plant group includes squashes, melons, and gourds like cucumbers, pumpkins, and luffas (that spongy fiber network you see in bath time sponges).

Grown as an annual and intolerant of frost, watermelon can be started indoors about three weeks before the last frost or directly sown when soil temperatures reach 70°F.

With over 1200 cultivars to choose from, it's best to find what grows well in your region.

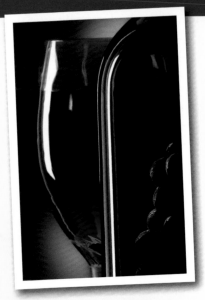

Filled with the scent of male pheromones

*A*T ONE TIME, IF MEN NEEDED TO REVIVE THEIR LIBIDO, THEY BEHEADED A partridge, poured the blood into a glass of water, and swallowed its heart. In the morning, they drank the blood concoction. Apparently, that went on for millennia. I think it's much easier to keep a corkscrew handy.

Records exist indicating that all species of wine grapes (*Vitis vinifera*) have been harvested since the Neolithic period, between 10,000 and 4,500 B.C., with aphrodisiac reference as early as the 8th century B.C., found on Babylonian cuneiform tablets.

During the Roman Empire, a Hippocras aphrodisiac was a well-loved drink: a red Burgundy wine fortified with various combinations of other aphrodisiac plants with benefits – ginger, cinnamon, cloves, and vanilla, as well as sugar. 'Twas a real mood setter.

WINE GRAPES

Family: Vitaceae

Type: Vine

Color: Green foliage, dark purple fruit

Harvest Period: Fall. Harvest occurs, on average, 120 days from flowering

Size: Vigorous grower to 10 to 20 feet each year

Soil: Sandy or clay loam

Exposure: Full sun

Watering: Occasional watering once established

pH: 6.5 to 8

Cold Hardiness Zone: 7 to 10

Origin: France

Nature gives us exactly what we need, right? If ever in doubt, think of Cabernet Sauvignon. In 17th century France, two neighboring vineyards, each field with a single parent, mingled and created a minor variety that turned out to be the most popular red wine grape ever, Cabernet Sauvignon, and a personal favorite of mine.

Why It Works: A Closer Look

Beyond the known health benefits of red wine, there are the sexual benefits. Most obvious is that a glass of red wine is known to reduce your inhibitions and generally put you in the mood. Red wine also has a scent that resembles a man's pheromones, thus exciting women.

Studies have found that alcohol temporarily raises the testosterone level of women (Sarkola et al. 2001). According to Dr. Andrew Weil, who published a 1994 study in *Nature*, "...small amounts can dramatically increase the libido. For women who lack sexual interest and desire, the treatment can be life-changing."

Drink responsibly, though; too much of this mood stimulator can have the opposite effect, and there's no fun in that!

GROWING TIPS

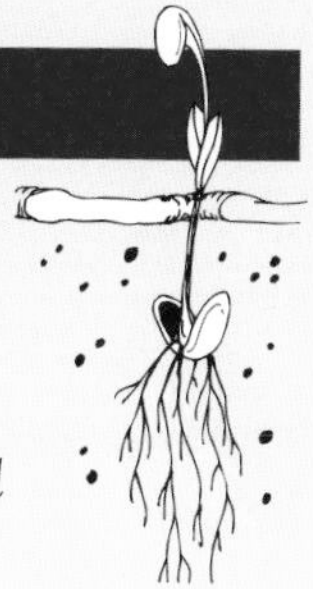

Considered a noble grape, Vitis vinifera *'Cabernet Sauvignon' can grow wherever red wine grapes grow.*

The grapes would need to be bottled and fermented. While making wine at home is a growing trend, feel free to purchase a bottle or two from your local store.

Hippocras
(a spiced wine)

Serves 6

Ahh, the marvels of modern – er, ancient – medicine. Back in the day, to keep things content, you may have been prescribed a cup of Hippocras, taken "during the hour of the bat." So set your clock to the evening hours, and share some aphrodisiac sips over pleasant conversation. You never know where the night will take you.

INGREDIENTS

1 bottle red wine (non-alcoholic wine or grape juice may be substituted)

1 cup honey

2 tablespoons cinnamon

2 tablespoons fresh grated ginger

1 tablespoon nutmeg

1 tablespoon cloves

1 tablespoon cardamom

1 tablespoon coriander

1 tablespoon cayenne

PREPARATION

Mix the spices together in a bowl and set aside. In a large pot, heat the wine or juice and honey to just below boiling.

Turn off the burner and add the spices to the wine. Allow to cool.

Pour the mixture into an airtight, glass container and set it in a cool, dark place for about a week. Strain the wine and return to the airtight container.

Let the wine mixture rest for about one month before drinking.

Unopened, the spiced wine will keep for a year. After opening, it will last about four days.

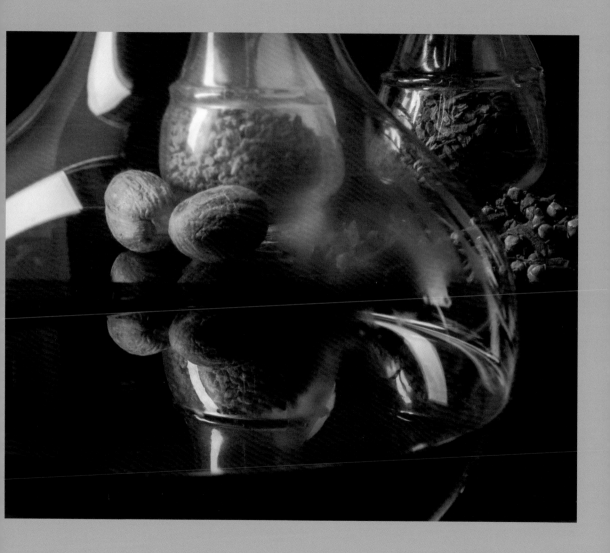

The Language of Flowers

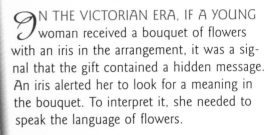

$\mathcal{I}$N THE VICTORIAN ERA, IF A YOUNG woman received a bouquet of flowers with an iris in the arrangement, it was a signal that the gift contained a hidden message. An iris alerted her to look for a meaning in the bouquet. To interpret it, she needed to speak the language of flowers.

Flowers do more than provide beauty and give joy; they can speak to you in place of a shy heart or declare a message as loud as a shout from the highest mountain.

Whether you're receiving the flowers, giving the arrangement, or even if you're picking them for yourself, you can give your flowers a voice. When the future queen of England, Kate Middleton, picked the flowers for her wedding bouquet, she made sure each one had a special meaning: lily-of-the-valley (return of happiness), sweet William (gallantry), hyacinth (constancy of lover), ivy (fidelity, marriage, wedded love and friendship) and myrtle (emblem of marriage and love). And she did it all in the tradition of white for purity. Even their wedding cake featured 17 different flower designs, each symbolizing a particular quality.

The precursor to the language of flowers was a form of love communication based on rhymes. It may trace its practice to the early Chinese dynasties, and later to Persia and the Turkish harems. In Turkey it was known as Selam, a kind of parlor trick – or more accurately, a harem game. For example, a young man would give his lady friend a pear (ermut), which in Turkish rhymes with umut, meaning "hope," The suitor would then add a phrase ending with the rhyming word, such as "Ermut, ver bize hir umut (Pear, give me some hope)."

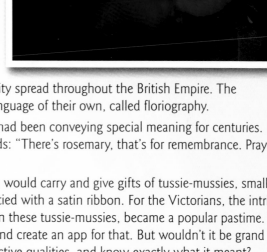

The Western world learned of this rhyming game in 1713 after Charles II of Sweden returned from a five-year exile in Turkey, where he lived at the Ottoman court. Thus, a new language of flowers started to take form, adapted from the Selam. And it spread from there.

Early on in Queen Victoria's reign, she became so enamored by the idea that its popularity spread throughout the British Empire. The Victorians, being inventive sorts, formulated a language of their own, called floriography.

Not that this was anything truly new. Flowers had been conveying special meaning for centuries. In Shakespeare's *Hamlet*, Ophelia speaks these words: "There's rosemary, that's for remembrance. Pray you, love, remember."

Since the late 15th century in England, women would carry and give gifts of tussie-mussies, small bouquets of flowers wrapped in a lace doily and tied with a satin ribbon. For the Victorians, the intrigue of secret messages, especially those hidden in these tussie-mussies, became a popular pastime. Perhaps we can put a modern day twist on this and create an app for that. But wouldn't it be grand to receive a single gardenia, with its scent and seductive qualities, and know exactly what it meant?

The language of flowers is certainly an expression to be preserved. Have you given a flower to someone you loved lately?

What the Flowers Say

Almond (flowering): Hope

Alstroemeria: Devotion and friendship

Alyssum: Worth beyond beauty

Amaranth: Affection

Amaryllis: Pride, beauty

Anemone: Forsaken

Apple Blossom: Good fortune

Artemisia: Dignity

Aster: Afterthought

Baby's Breath: Everlasting love

Basil: Best wishes

Bachelor's Button: Celibacy

Bellflower: Gratitude

Calla Lily: Beauty

Camellia (Red): I love you

Camellia (White): Loveliness

Carnation (solid): Pride and beauty, fascination

Carnation (striped): Refusal

Chrysanthemum (yellow): Disappointment

Coreopsis: Always cheerful

Crocus: Youthful gladness

Cyclamen: It's over, goodbye

Daffodil: Unrequited Love

Dahlia: Instability

Daisy: Innocence, attachment

Edelweiss: Cleanliness

Forget-me-not: True love

Foxglove: Insincerity

French Honeysuckle: Rustic beauty

French Marigold: Jealousy

Gardenia: Secret love

Gladiola: Sincerity

Geranium: Melancholy

Goldenrod: Precaution

Heather (pink): Good luck

Hibiscus: Delicate beauty

Hollyhock: Ambition

Honeysuckle: Devoted affection

Hyssop: Cleanliness

Iris: Signals there is a message in the bouquet

Jasmine: Amiability

Lantana: Rigor

Larkspur: Lightness

Laurel: Glory

Lemon Blossoms: Fidelity

Lilac: First sign of love

Lily: Purity of heart

Lily (white): Purity and sweetness

Lily (orange): Hatred

Lily of the Valley: Return of happiness

Lotus: Eloquence

Love-in-a-Mist: Perplexity

Lupine: Imagination

Magnolia: Love of nature

Marigold: Cruelty or jealousy

Marjoram: Blushes

Mint: Virtue
Morning Glory: Love in vain
Nasturtium: Patriotism
Orange Blossom: Marriage and fruitfulness
Orchid: Beauty
Oleander: Beware
Orange Blossoms: Purity
Pansy: Messenger of love
Periwinkle (blue): Early friendship
Periwinkle (white): Pleasures of memory
Phlox: Unanimity
Poppy (red): Consolation
Peony: Happy marriage
Ranunculus: You are radiant with charms
Rosemary: Remembrance
Rudbeckia: Justice
Sweet Pea: Goodbye
Sunflower: Adoration
Spearmint: Warm affections
Red Tulips: Delectation of love
Rhododendron: Strength
Snapdragon: Presumption
Snowdrop: Hope
Star of Bethlehem: Purity
Sunflower: Adoration
Thistle: Austerity
Thyme: Activity
Trumpet Flower: Fame
Tuberose: Dangerous pleasure
Tulip (red): Declaration of love
Tulip (variegated): Beautiful eyes
Veronica: Fidelity

Violet (blue): Faithfulness
Violet (yellow): Happiness,
Yellow Daylilies: Coquetry, flirtation
Zinnia (burgundy): Lasting affection
Zinnia (mixed): Thoughts of an absent friend
Queen Anne's Lace: Fantasy

The Meaning of Certain Rose Colors and Types

Coral: Desire
Black: Death
Lavender: Enhancement
Pink: Admiration, appreciation, grace, happiness,
   thanks, grace, gentleness, happiness, and please
   believe me
Pink, dark: Appreciation, gratitude, thank you
Pink, light: Admiration, gentleness, grace,
   gladness, joy, sweetness, and sympathy
Orange: Desire and enthusiasm
Peach: Let's get together
Red: Passionate love, beauty, courage, respect,
   and congratulations
Red, dark: Unconscious beauty
Red and White given together: Unity
Red and yellow blends: Jovial and happy feelings
White: Purity, innocence, silence, secrecy,
   reverence, youthfulness, I am worth of you
Yellow: Contentment, delight, friendship, joy, the
   promise of a new beginning, I care
Yellow with a red tip: Falling in love

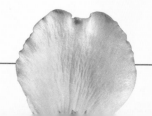

GLOSSARY

Adaptogens: a unique group of herbal ingredients thought to improve the health of your adrenal system, the system that's in charge of managing your body's hormonal response to stress. They're called adaptogens because of their unique ability to "adapt" their function according to your body's specific needs.

Allicin: a compound found in garlic that can improve blood flow to the sexual organs.

Allopathic medicine: the practice of traditional Western medicine, using drugs or surgery to diagnose or suppress a disease; as distinguished from the approaches used by homeopathy or naturopathy.

Amino acids: organic compounds that play a vital role in normal sexual function and will help increase levels of nitric oxide in the body.

Anandamide: one of the three "love drug" chemicals that stimulate the pleasure centers. The other two are phenylethylamine (PEA) and tryptophan.

Anethole: found in aniseed; stimulates sexual drive by inducing effects similar to testosterone; helps prepare the female body for childbirth; increases breast-milk production in nursing mothers.

Aphrodisiac: any substance that restores or increases sexual desire or functioning.

Aphrodite: Greek goddess of love and beauty.

The Arabian Nights: a collection of magical tales compiled and translated into Arabic during the Islamic Golden Age (mid-8th century to the 13th century) from stories and folk tales of South and West Asia. It includes references to cardamom, coriander and other foods as aphrodisiacs.

Arginine, also L-arginine: a vasodilator amino acid; a precursor to nitric oxide. Found in some medicated creams and gels which, when applied to the genitals, can increase arousal.

Ayurvedic Medicine: India's 5,000-year-old Science of Life; one of the world's oldest medical systems, focusing on herbal compounds and special diets and based on five basic types of human temperament and characteristics, called doshas. It has its origins in India's ancient Vedic culture. Ayurveda is considered an alternative or complementary medicine in the West.

Aztecs: the native civilization in Mesoamerica when the Spanish arrived in the 16th century (see Montezuma).

Bacchus: believed by the Romans to have introduced the grape to mankind; the equivalent to the Greek god Dionysus, god of revelry, wine and fertility.

Benzyl Acetate: along with jasmone, this chemical creates jasmine's essential oils, which help the body relax and relieve stress.

Boron: a mineral found in food (such as honey) that increases estrogen production in women.

Capsaicin: the active component in cayenne and other chili peppers, sometimes sold in the form of an extract.

Chrysin: a chemical found in food (such as honey) that improves testosterone production in men.

Crocin: a natural carotenoid chemical and potent anti-oxidant found in saffron threads.

Cineole: a chemical found in cardamom that increases blood flow.

Cinnamaldehyde: the essential oil derived from the leaves, flower buds and bark of the cinnamon tree. It acts as a warming agent that increases circulation in the pelvic area.

Citrulline: an amino acid that not only benefits the cardiovascular and immune systems, but also enables the body to relax and expand blood vessels, thus facilitating the libido. Found in the rind of watermelon.

Dioscorides: Greek physician (c. 40-90 A.D.) who created the first system of botanical terminology and the leading pharmacological text for 1,600 years.

Doctrine of Signatures: the philosophy that the design or appearance of every plant gives clues to its purpose.

Dopamine: the neurotransmitter associated with the pleasure system of the brain.

Essential fatty acids: needed for the production of hormones (testosterone), reproductive function, fertility and healthy libido.

Estragole: found in anise and fennel; may increase sexual drive.

Estrogen: a female steroid sex hormone produced by the ovaries and in lesser degree by the male testes.

Flavonoid: a chemical that helps promote blood vessel health by stimulating blood flow.

Folic Acid: a nutrient helpful in stimulating your metabolism, boosting histamine production necessary to reach orgasm in both sexes.

Alan Hirsch, M.D., F.A.C.P.: founder and neurological director of the Smell & Taste Treatment and Research Foundation in Chicago.

Jasmone: along with benzyl acetate, this chemical creates jasmine's essential oils, which help the body relax and relieve stress.

Kama Sutra: ancient Indian Hindu text thought to be the earliest work on human sexual behavior, the nature of love and the many pleasures of human life.

Montezuma: leader of the Aztec nation when the Spanish Conquistadors arrived in Mesoamerica. He was knowledgeable about local aphrodisiacs, like chocolate, vanilla and cayenne.

N-acyl-ethanolamines (NAEs): delivers the necessary energy required for a healthy sex life, by uplifting the mood for sex.

Nitric oxide synthase (NOS): a vasodilator enzyme thought to be primarily responsible for the mechanism of erection.

Omega-3 fatty acid: an essential fatty acid that assists metabolism.

The Perfumed Garden: a 15th century Arabic sex manual and work of erotic literature.

Phenylethylamine (PEA): stimulates the same hormone (oxytocin) your body releases during sex and sparks dopamine production in the brain.

Phenylpropene: a type of organic compound found in fennel, licorice and star anise with an aroma and taste that can increase arousal.

Pheromone: a chemical that influences the behavior of other animals of the same species, often for attracting the opposite sex.

Phthalide: an organic chemical found in celery that acts as a vasodilator.

Phytoestrogens: estrogen-like chemicals that are found in plant foods (like fennel and coriander), believed to stimulate sexual desire in women and help regulate hormones.

Pliny the Elder (Gaius Plinius Secundus): Roman author, naturalist and philosopher (c. 23-79 A.D.) who established the model for encyclopedias with his book of natural science.

Potassium: a mineral that helps erections by improving circulation.

Priapus: Greek god of animal and vegetable fertility and male generative power. Always shown with a huge and permanently erect phallus.

Testosterone: a steroid hormone that plays a key role in male development. Low testosterone in males can coontribute to erectile dysfunction. Testosterone is also present, but less so, in females; however, low levels contribute to a lowering of libido in both sexes.

Tryptophan: one of the three "love drug" chemicals that stimulate the pleasure centers. The other two are phenyl-ethylamine (PEA) and anandamide (AEA).

Vasodilator: a substance capable of dilating or opening blood vessels.

Vitamin A: maintains the sexual hormone function in men and women and keeps skin from becoming dry.

Vitamin B complex: increases levels of testosterone and fuels the sex drive in both men and women; keeps the thyroid, nervous system and adrenal glands content.

Vitamin B6 and folate (B9): helpful in stress reduction and better testosterone production; can boost orgasm and arousal.

Vitamin C: keeps the skin smooth, helps prevent miscar-riages, keeps sperm from clinging together in immobile clusters, and enables more intense, longer lasting orgasms.

Vitamin E: found in nuts, seeds, whole grains, fruits and vegetables; helps the blood carry oxygen; offsets the loss of estrogen in post-menopausal women; keeps testoster-one from breaking down in men.

Vitamin P: a mid-20th century term for flavonoids.

Yin and Yang: a traditional Chinese medicine concept that promotes balance between opposites: Yin (heat, positivity, masculinity) and Yang (cold, negativity, femininity).

Zinc: essential for the production of testosterone; low levels may reduce sperm count, potency, sex drive and long-term sexual health; insufficient zinc in women may cause dryness of the vagina.

INDEX

RECIPES

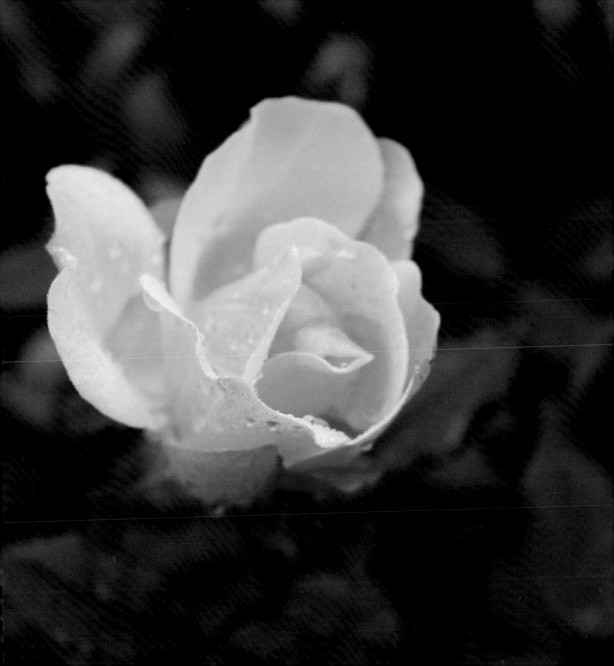

ACKNOWLEDGMENTS

When my publisher, Paul Kelly, first asked me to write *Plants with Benefits*, I blushed. It's not as if I limit my thoughts to those of a Puritan. On the contrary. It's just that the idea came out of left field, it seemed. To get through the telephone conversation, I had to imagine Paul as a priest behind the screen in a confessional. It worked. We ran with the book idea. Paul is amazing to work with, and I'm truly honored he had the faith in me to write this book.

Working with Paul meant I also got to work with St. Lynn's Press editor Cathy Dees. Paul describes Cathy as a word doctor, and indeed she is. Her prescriptions were always taken, making me feel better and my writing look good. I describe her as a lifelong friend, even though we only just met prior to starting the book. We both still have a long life ahead. She'll be there, somewhere, in my life going forward.

With Cathy came two summer interns, Chloe Wertz and Annamarie Mickey, and later, Claire Stetzer and Allison Keene. It was a privilege discovering with them. I have no doubt that lavender and licorice now line their spice rack.

To my delight, I also had the good fortune to work with Holly Rosborough, Art Director at St. Lynn's Press. I think Holly should be called the "Smile Director," because that is what I do when I see her work. Holly has the artistic ability to make anything I say look just a little bit better.

In researching many of these plants, I often found that I questioned some of the information. During those times, I called upon my dear friends and go-to horticulturists, Mark Weathington, Tim Alderton and Chris Glenn from the JC Raulston Arboretum, and John Buettner, who never seems to be without an answer. I'm not sure how I got so lucky to have them in my life, but it is certainly made the better for it.

I'm more apt to want to prepare food if I can grow it in the garden. Many of the recipes in the book were contributed by my dear friend Carolyn Binder, of Cowlick Cottage Farm. She likes to spend her weekends experimenting in the kitchen. I benefit from her discoveries and I hope you will, too. Much of what Carolyn prepares includes fresh picks of the day from her garden.

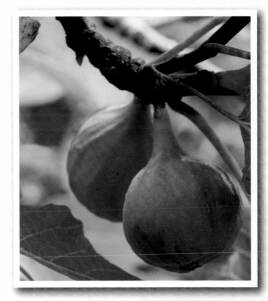

Many of the photos in the book were styled, photographed and edited by David Spain and Ken Gergle. I don't believe the book could have become what it is without their vision and talent. David is the owner of Moss and Stone Gardens and Ken is an award-winning photographer whose work has been in some of the nation's leading magazines accompanying feature stories, and in ad copy for several Fortune 100 companies. I feel very fortunate that our paths have crossed. Ken and I are collaborating on other works.

And finally...before I could say yes to the book schedule, I told St. Lynn's Press I needed to check with my husband and make sure he had my back to help with the kids. He did. As usual. My life has been enriched beyond words by my husband of 25 years, David Philbrook, and our three children, Lara Rose, Lily Ana and Michael Aster. After all this time, David has never questioned my curiosity, and even seems to indulge me. The kids put up with me, most of the time. I'm happy with that.

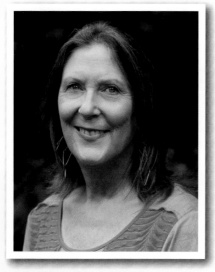

HELEN YOEST is a curious gardener – curious about plants, soil, design, and how others use these to create their gardens at home. She is also curious about what plants do for us today in the here and now, but also about their history and lore. Plants have a colorful past.

As an award winning freelance writer and garden stylist, Helen has traveled the world visiting public and private gardens so she can step into the dream that was once just an imagination. Her work has appeared in *Country Gardens, Better Homes and Gardens, Martha Stewart Living, Carolina Gardener,* and many others, including her work as the national gardening expert for Answers.com. Helen is also the author of *Gardening with Confidence, 50 Ways to Add Style for Personal Creativity.*

Helen curates garden art, serves on the board of the JC Raulston Arboretum, is past Regional Representative of the Garden Conservancy Open Days tour, and is an honorary member of Pi Alpha Xi, the national honor society for floriculture, landscape horticulture and ornamental horticulture.

Helen lives in Raleigh, N.C., tending to her half-acre wildlife habitat, her husband, and their three beautiful children. She opens her garden annually to the public.

Visit Helen at her popular blog, gardeningwithconfidence.com and at plantswithbenefits.com.